NAVIGATING
SHITSTORMS

LIZ LONG

NAVIGATING
SHITSTORMS

How to Find Your True Path

When Life Gets Rough

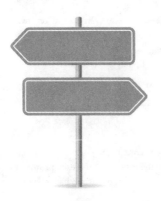

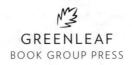

GREENLEAF
BOOK GROUP PRESS

Published by Greenleaf Book Group Press
Austin, Texas
www.gbgpress.com

Distributed by Greenleaf Book Group

For ordering information or special discounts for bulk purchases, please contact Greenleaf Book Group at PO Box 91869, Austin, TX 78709, 512.891.6100.

Design and composition by Greenleaf Book Group and Teresa Muñiz
Cover design by Greenleaf Book Group and Teresa Muñiz

Publisher's Cataloging-in-Publication data is available.

Print ISBN: 979-8-88645-072-9

eBook ISBN: 979-8-88645-073-6

To offset the number of trees consumed in the printing of our books, Greenleaf donates a portion of the proceeds from each printing to the Arbor Day Foundation. Greenleaf Book Group has replaced over 50,000 trees since 2007.

Printed in the United States of America on acid-free paper

23 24 25 26 27 28 29 30   10 9 8 7 6 5 4 3 2 1

First Edition

To Lynda, who walks beside me still as I brave my life journey with as much intrinsic courage as I can muster.

Respair (n): the return of hope after a long period of despair

Contents

Prologue

It's November 22, 2020, and I'm not traveling for pleasure. I'm not about to embark on a vacation. I'm on my way for a self-imposed stay at a . . . I'm not sure what to call it. A place, I guess. When I was organizing to leave and letting a few people know, I got out of naming it by sending them the link to the website. "This is where I'm going. I'll let you know when I'm out," I said. Some might call it rehab or a treatment center. Joking around, my best friend and I called it "the puzzle factory" and "The Place for broken toys." It's kind of irrelevant anyway. I mean, who cares what it's called? It's not like someone is *making* me go. I haven't been committed. There was no intervention.

I booked a first-class pod for my journey. Never have I done that. It's an indulgence afforded by the accumulation of 350,000 air miles. Toronto's Pearson International Airport is one of the busiest airports in North America. I thought I'd feel special when I was called to board before everyone else, but I didn't. I am, however, grateful. I've always dreamed of traveling first class. It was a totally decadent thing to do. I did it because I'm so exhausted, all I want to do is sleep all day. Every day actually, but especially on this flight. The biggest reason though, the real truth if you will, is that I'm in this first-class pod because I desperately don't want to become known as the "airplane crier." Last, but not least, this pod keeps me truly six feet away from any sneezy super-spreaders even though a voice in my head sometimes suggests that dying of COVID-19 wouldn't be the worst thing. That's the voice that makes me cry.

My pod is fully equipped with my very own big screen TV, a laptop shelf, a blanket, a pillow as big as my own, two water bottles, a bag of pretzels . . . and a seat that turns into a bed! Sleep might be possible after all.

What have I done?

This decision bears no resemblance to drunk-booking an all-inclusive trip with a relative stranger. Or random purchases from Facebook ads. Nope. Not even a little bit.

I'm such an idiot. I completely overreacted. Again.

What do I have to be so depressed about anyway? I'm pathetic. And weak. The people there will have real issues, serious problems.

But at least I'll be living. And maybe I'll even learn to like myself. Wouldn't it be great to be happy?

But what if it doesn't work? What if it's too hard? What if I just can't do it? What am I gonna do if this place doesn't fix me? Huh? What then?

Without warning my peripheral vision catches something odd.

What the hell?

I turn and stare at the passenger across the aisle. I see a full-face plastic shield with a hoodie pulled tight and the string knotted to prevent even the slightest opening. Through the clear shield I see not one, but two cloth face masks, one on top of the other, and wrap-around protective glasses.

How can they see through all that plastic?

Barely a square inch of skin is visible. A tight turtleneck reaches up to meet the mask. Hands are concealed in blue latex gloves tucked snugly under the cuffs of long sleeves. Socks are pulled up and over pants to prevent any exposed ankle skin. The final layer, the grand cape of fortification, is a yellow paper surgeon's gown. Protection to the max. It looks like an astronaut! The only things I can see are eyes.

Holy shit! What is wrong with them? It's not an apocalypse for crying out loud.

Or is it? Am I missing something?

Ashamed by my invasive curiosity and judgment, I look away before I'm caught, and like a heavy blanket, another layer of fear settles over me.

Serves you right for never watching the news. You're so stupid. And now you're exposed!

I have no protection. I didn't bring the right armor. Well, other than a single mask and an old purse-size bottle of fruity hand sanitizer, which is a few years old, so any actual disinfectant properties have probably long expired.

It's all so completely inadequate. Like you.

My eyes start to well up. Again. The problem isn't wine and Netflix every night. My only problem is the crying. That and wanting to die.

Before I decided to go to The Place, I was an average human holding it all together, like a lot of us do. It wasn't like I was idle or passive about the holding either. I tried to feel better. I did put effort in. I'm a doer, so I tried to *do* all the things that everyone said would make it better. And I think I tried pretty damn hard. I joined the gym and showed up regularly. I spent time with friends. I vacationed. I drank. I went to therapy. I laughed. I partied. And I worked. A lot.

Then, disillusioned by the lack of industry integrity and the antics of my unethical colleagues, I walked away from a very lucrative real estate career. But shit kept happening. And piling up. A shoulder injury, a heartbreaking disappointment and subsequent fallout with a business partner who was like my daughter.

On and on it went. A reneged promise to propose by my boyfriend. An extra twenty pounds. My only sibling was estranged, and my dearest friend of fifty-two years dumped me with a text. It was monumental shit, inconsequential shit, and everything in between—from the ominous responsibility to fix some major problems that people I loved were having to a shortage of critical firewood for my winter woodstove. Then COVID-19 cases surfaced in my mom's long-term care residence and prevented me from visiting, which, to be honest, was a huge relief. But that relief also brought immense judgment and shame.

Some of it surprised me, but mostly I'd come to expect it. Some of it I didn't deserve, but mostly I knew that I did. Occasionally I could handle it, but mostly I was in over my head. The pandemic collapsed my new business launch. I embraced gratitude. I focused on the fact that so many other people had things way worse than me. I felt overwhelmed anyway.

As the shit pile got bigger and bigger, I did more therapy. I meditated daily for weeks and then I'd forget. I had a lovely roof over my head and food was plentiful. I ate well. I ate junk. I ate too much. I didn't eat enough. I was hungry for something I couldn't identify. Starving, in fact. As I drank wine and binge-watched shows on Netflix, I ruminated about the past, felt browbeaten by the present, and was completely dismayed about the future.

Bringing my eighty-two-year-old dad with me, I relocated to a remote lakeside house several hours away from my friends and family. For the first time in my entire life, my world became quiet and still. Space emerged. Nobody needed me. A vast, unending emptiness arrived, and I saw the nothingness in every direction I looked. It enveloped me. Trapped and unable to fill the void, all the experiences and emotions that I'd locked deep inside of me for years began to leak out, and I cracked. Just like a modern-day Humpty Dumpty. I started buying wine by the case—arguably for efficiency's sake 'cause it's a bit of a trek into town, but one time I made it in pajamas. Shhh. Not only did the world no longer need me, the voice in my head also told me that I

didn't need me. Uncaring, I started lying to people I loved and fanta-
sizing daily about how to orchestrate my demise.

I became a "town crier." Don't get the wrong idea, I wasn't out there
yelling "hear-ye, hear-ye." I was literally crying. Unprovoked and in
front of innocent people. And not the dainty whimpering, single-tear-
rolling-down-the-cheek kind of crying. Oh no. What was happening to
me was the red-eyed, nose-dripping, sputtering kind of crying. I wasn't
fit for public consumption.

In my defense, I did hold it together for a long time, well into my fifties, in fact, and through a lot of shit. A lot of nasty shitstorms. But when
I couldn't reset my Netflix account, I said to myself, "Houston, we have
a problem." That was my tipping point. Netflix deprivation was about to
kill me. I can't be the only one. I mean, you can relate, right?

I always knew I was collateral damage as a child. That was just part of
my life, and I didn't give it much thought. In 1968, Lynda White, my
favorite aunt and babysitter, disappeared. At the age of nineteen, in her
first year at the University of Western Ontario, she vanished. I was six.

I witnessed firsthand the devastation that the "not knowing if she
was alive or dead" brought to our family. For five excruciating years of
my childhood, this angst consumed us. We endured divorces, financial crisis, and the death of my baby sister. My maternal grandmother's
grief-driven psychosis and my grandfather's debilitating stroke
required my mother to step into the role of managing police detectives
and private investigators—and to completely check out of parenting.
The cherry on top was when we moved in with my grandparents, and I
was given Lynda's bedroom. So many people suffered, but two children
were trapped in the front-line turmoil. I was one of those children. I
wouldn't know for most of my life what that really meant.

The discovery of Lynda's body in 1973 only led to more conjecture and unanswerable questions. My remaining years at home brought random evidence discoveries, regular visits from psychics with new insights, and retiring detectives stopping by to tell us they were not giving up.

My coping mechanisms were not unique. The new and different behaviors I adopted, along with my beliefs about the world, had one consistent and laser-focused purpose: to protect myself. From everything. It became second nature for me to avoid getting snatched. I braced myself for people I loved to abandon me. I knew my needs were not important. I locked the overwhelming helplessness deep inside and did everything within my power to be self-reliant and shield myself from further hurt of any kind whatsoever.

My teenage years brought some wonky parental rules, as you might imagine. My mother projected her fear onto me, and I rebelled with a vengeance. At the same time, I became an expert at personal safety (you know, just in case). I armored up, as I was launched out into the world for good at the age of eighteen.

But it didn't end there. For the next three decades, a constant stream of events unfolded that continued to bring my family's unrelenting pain to the surface. These events came in the form of emerging DNA technology, new developments in crime software, sensational TV shows, and best-selling books about unsolved murders—and the victims' families. I was aware of it all, but I honestly didn't think that it had anything to do with my present-day struggles. Boy, was I ever wrong!

I had no idea that one day, because Lynda disappeared, I wouldn't be able to reset my Netflix account and I would end up in The Place. I also had no idea that my coping mechanisms from childhood—the things that kept me safe and relatively sane for so long—were responsible for my shitty life and would eventually fail me entirely.

You might think this is the kind of story where I go to a place, heal my childhood shit, magically live happily ever after, and then write about it. That's not what happened. Not only did my road trip have sizeable bumps and detours, I was also listening to a very shitty playlist in my head. It's been fifty-four years without answers—for me or my family.

We all miss her.

As of this writing, Lynda's case remains one of the longest unsolved murders in Canada.

Introduction

Full disclosure—it took me fifty-eight years to figure out most of my shit. Fifty-eight.

And that's okay. I can't change it, so it might as well be okay. I still don't have everything sorted out, but I've learned things firsthand, things that I believe will help you, too.

You should also know I don't have a medical degree. I'm not a therapist. And I'm not a self-help guru. I'm just an ordinary person. Sure, I wrote this self-help book, but at the same time, there's not a doubt in my mind that I will always need to "self-help" myself every time life throws me a curve.

Let's face it: Shit happens. It happens to everyone, and children are not immune. And it happens throughout our lives. But the thing is, life's too short not to feel happy and fulfilled. If you're one of the lucky people who magically escaped any negative experiences in your childhood and are living a blissful life as an adult, you probably don't need to read this book. But maybe you're just curious about my story. Or maybe you've already reconciled with what happened in your childhood and as you're reading may find similarities to your own journey.

If, however, you're feeling lost or wondering about how you got *here*, if *here* for you is lacking in any way, it's my heartfelt intention for the following pages to bring you *respair*. Respair is an old word that I recently came across. Dating back to 1425, it means "the return of hope after a long period of despair."[1]

You see, many months after checking myself into The Place for depression, there was still something missing—an elusive lens through which my life would finally make sense—so I gave it a name. It's called Victimtown. You may think you've never been there, but I can say with certainty that you have. We all have. If you're skeptical, maybe just skip straight to any of the chapters in Part 2. You can go back and read how it all starts later.

Victimtown, and all the places that exist there, changed the way I thought about our world. Victimtown offers a fresh perspective about the voices in our head. This is pretty important stuff because our inner dialogue forms the foundation of our mental health. You may not think of yourself as a victim. I sure didn't. And I can be stubborn. So, it was a slow and very begrudging journey that eventually led me to this truth: To varying degrees, every one of us is a victim of our childhood.

While we can't absolutely stop bad things from happening, this book will show you a fresh way of looking at life. It's an introduction to another voice, one that will help you navigate Victimtown and (when you're ready) find your way out and be on your way to Freedomville. It'll also help you navigate shitstorms throughout your life.

I ran smack into the realization that my childhood coping mechanisms were never meant to be permanent. I discovered that spending a certain amount of time in Victimtown is not only unavoidable, but also it can offer unparalleled gifts. And that's what eventually got the job done for me.

Life is dynamic—always moving, always changing. It takes great courage to face your wounds in Victimtown. So, if or when you find yourself back there, it just means you're ready to heal another wound and learn another lesson. We always get to choose. What playlist are you going to listen to when life gets rough? Which voice in your head will you believe and sing along with? It's an important question because the song you're singing to yourself, the tune you're humming, well, that's going to lead you to either Victimtown or Freedomville.

I hope you'll keep turning the pages and know that you're not alone.

Liz Long, Sechelt, BC, Canada, 2022

PART 1

Childhood

CHAPTER 1

It All Starts in Childhood

We are all born for love, it is the
principle of existence and its only end.
—*Benjamin Disraeli*

When I arrived at The Place, I thought all my struggles were because I was fundamentally deficient as a human. I mean, I knew there were events from my past that I would probably need to unpack and reconcile, as just about everyone has some of those. But it was more than that. I believed that, at my core, I was flawed. I thought I was born that way. Once again, I was wrong. This time I was glad about it.

You Were Born with an Open Heart

Every single human is born as pure love. Nothing else, just love. Sure, it's a corny statement, but I believe it's true. When we're born, we're vulnerable in every way possible. In spite of being dependent for our very survival, we have complete trust in the entire world. Why? Because our minds and hearts are free of impurities and debris— untainted by pain, disappointment, or hurt. We've not yet learned the one thing that changes everything—fear.

With our hearts strong and wide open, we give and receive immense amounts of love. We are whole. Our perfection is uncontested as we love everything about ourselves. We don't judge or compare. We honor our intrinsic human value. And we honor everyone else's too. Without limits or conditions, we believe we are worthy of our unique place in the world. We don't question it.

Wouldn't it be great if we stayed that way?

Yes. And no. Although it does sound lovely, the reality is that our most valuable lessons occur only after we lose our way. It's like the saying, "You don't know what you've got till it's gone." Our struggle to find our way back to our hearts is what enables us to truly appreciate it when we do return home. To Freedomville.

Starting with cries and facial expressions, then pointing and grunt-ing, we ask for everything we need and want. From there, we grow into toddlers with a boundless attitude of curiosity as we begin to explore our world. We offer our love to everyone and everything. Instinctively, we follow our hearts' desires without care or consideration of what anyone thinks. Joy is our unapologetic mission. As we learn to use our words, we continue to expect only love in return. Our courage is intrinsic. We joyfully take chances and try new things. We view our mistakes and failures with gratitude for the lessons learned, and we use them to spur us on to greater achievements.

All humans begin life full of peace, love, freedom, and joy. This is our natural set point and part of our hearts' DNA. As we begin to interact more with the world, our new experiences bring a myriad of new feelings.

> All humans begin life full of
> peace, love, freedom, and joy.

Feelings Are a Big Deal

Unfortunately, more often than not, emotional intelligence is learned, developed, and strengthened by trial and error. Education about feelings sure wasn't in the curriculum when I was at school. Nor did my parents teach it intentionally or well. But teach it they did, as all parents do because children are incredibly perceptive. As kids try to make sense of emotions and feelings, it's probably a good thing that they have no way to appreciate the monumental proportions of the task. I think there are a gazillion adults out there still struggling to make sense of emotions, their own and others', which shows how hard they are to get a handle on.

Lots of us have trouble naming our feelings. I get it. Talking about feelings can be uncomfortable for anyone, parents included. In fairness to them, it's unreasonable to expect anyone to teach something they don't understand or appreciate. We learned early on that we were vulnerable when we expressed our feelings.

We also learned that feelings are subject to judgment. While some feelings were okay to express, others were not. Children are very susceptible to influence. Under the control of our caregivers, some of us learned that certain feelings should be avoided at all costs. We encountered this at home, in school, or playing in the neighborhood. It wasn't just negative feelings that we learned to avoid. Sometimes, too much joy was deemed inappropriate and, therefore, unacceptable. Such bullshit. When I was growing up, boys were taught that it was wrong to cry. Some of us were even *told* to ignore our feelings. We heard directives like—

"Stop dwelling on it."

"You're not really hurt."

"There's no need to be *that* upset."

"Stop being such a baby."

"Big boys don't cry."

"Don't be such a scaredy cat."

"You're being way too sensitive."

"Stop crying. RIGHT NOW!"

Some well-intentioned parents respond to their children's painful feelings by saying all kinds of things to help them avoid discomfort. When a child's pain is internalized by a parent, the parent often diminishes it to protect themselves. In doing so, they rob the child of their own emotional education. It's not done maliciously; parents who love their children really are all doing their best.

The healthy functioning of feelings, however, is vital. Our feelings are a guidance system of sorts. We could even call it our built-in Happiness GPS. Whether we want it or not, it's part of the package we're all born with. Everyone has the capacity to feel. What a beautiful thing! But there is one caveat: When we don't understand the purpose of our feelings, when we're not capable of fully embracing our feelings, we lose out on the intel. Our Happiness GPS malfunctions. Not learning emotional intelligence as kids inadvertently introduces us to many of the places in Victimtown when, inevitably, shit happens.

Our feelings are a guidance system of sorts,
like a built-in Happiness GPS.

CHAPTER 2

Shit Happens

You know those bumper stickers where it says,
"Shit Happens, And Then You Die"? They should
have them where it says, "Shit Happens, And Then
You Live," because that's really the truth of it.

—*Anna Nicole Smith*

C hildhood is when we form relationships for the first time. We learn how to be with ourselves, other people, and the world at large. We begin the monumental task of interpreting what our world is all about, what everything *means*. Then we have to determine how we fit into that world. All children have to do this.

Adverse Childhood Experiences

The Place taught me that early traumatic events are called Adverse Childhood Experiences by psychologists, or ACEs for short. The numbers are staggering.

ACEs are common. About 61 percent of adults surveyed across 25 states reported they had experienced at least one type of ACE before age 18, and nearly 1 in 6 reported they had experienced four or more types of ACEs.[1]

Some children dealt with benign incidents, while others were subjected to horrific situations. Our childhood traumas can be plotted on a long spectrum ranging from trivial to tragic, but that's not the important part. No matter where our experiences fall on this spectrum, the fact that we were *on* the spectrum means that as adults, we likely need to unpack some shit.

Big Ts and Little ts

Traumas can be divided loosely into two categories. The *big T* traumas include war, accidents, death, threats to life, and safety issues. *Little t* traumas are the chronic stressors like verbal and emotional abuse, nonattentive parents, and bullying. These events, when experienced as a one-off, are often just a part of life without a long-lasting impact. But when a *little t* happens repetitively, they add up to a *big T*. Trivial can turn into tragic over time. Being bullied is one example. Each time it happens, it may be manageable. But when we're bullied day after day after day, the result can be the same as if we were severely assaulted and hospitalized for weeks.

According to Dr. Bruce D. Perry, a renowned brain development and trauma expert, it's not only major traumatic events that affect us. Unpredictable stress at home and the lack of control that goes with it can also have long-lasting effects. Additionally, Perry states, "neglect is as toxic as trauma." Neglect is a heading with many components. We also lose our way when our needs aren't met often enough, consistently enough, or at the right times. If we didn't get the attention, reassurance, guidance, hugs, or food when we needed it, we suffered. And in that suffering, we learned to see the world through a lens of fear.[2]

Some children may react to something seemingly trivial in a way that's very detrimental to their mental health. Each of us has different tolerances and sensitivities. A *little t* for one person could be tragic for another. One *little t* can cause a child to lose their way, depending on their response. The determining factor is how we figure it out—more specifically, in the meaning we attach to the event. Many of us assume that *big Ts* are way harder to deal with, but I would say, not necessarily. As individuals, we're qualified to make the judgment of what's better or worse only when it relates to ourselves, never about how it is for anyone else. It's not a competition, anyway. There will always be someone who had a worse childhood than us as well as someone who didn't have it nearly as bad. That's not the point.

If you think what happened to you wasn't bad enough or is completely unrelated to your issues as an adult (as I did), you may be surprised and skeptical (as I was) to learn this: The factor that bears the most impact on our future is not what actually happened to us. The critical element is how, as children, we responded to it. I'm not saying that the severity of our traumas isn't relevant. It absolutely is. But the severity isn't always the most influential component in how it affects us for the rest of our lives. Our responses, the ways we internalized the ACEs we lived through, and the meanings we came up with are what's most predictive of our internal dialogue and the subsequent coping mechanisms we developed and carried into our adult lives.

What determines our future is not what actually
happened to us, but rather, how we responded to it.

Connecting the Dots

From the time we're born, we're on a mission to interpret and understand how the world works. Babies and children are like sponges. They miss nothing. Using the human senses available to them, children set out to comprehend the world.

Our brains must make the connection between the event and its meaning so we can plan and anticipate how we'll respond in the future. But there's a problem. Our brains can't stop until they come up with a meaning. Anything will do. A meaning that's highly unlikely or even ridiculous is better than no meaning at all. Only after acquiring a meaning can our brain relax knowing its work is done.

In the beginning, we asked lots of questions and, every now and then, answers or explanations were offered to us. Some of us were expressly told why or how something happened and exactly what it meant. Provided by a parent, teacher, coach, or even another kid, these explanations were, however, only one person's interpretation. Often unaware of the ramifications, the adults in our world who offered an explanation sometimes provided a meaning that was inaccurate, inadequate, or incomplete. Sometimes we believed them, sometimes we didn't. Sometimes what the adults told us was helpful and healthy for us; sometimes it wasn't.

Many adults were unable or unwilling to even try. When the questions became too hard to ask or there was nobody willing to answer or we didn't believe the explanation we were given, we were left with only our imaginations and our fears to come up with a story that would adequately fill in the blanks and explain what it all meant. This was the only way we could come to grips with whatever occurred. Our brains demanded it. Unfortunately, almost all of the time, this resulted in a shitty belief or three.

It's a normal part of childhood development for our brains to operate with this fill-in-the-blank mandate. The majority of the stories we told ourselves as children have little resemblance to the truth. We might not even remember the details of those long-ago made-up stories, but they got into our bones. Worse, the stories got into our hearts.

> Our brains must determine a meaning;
> any meaning will do.

Devised to explain something bad that happened (an ACE), the meanings and stories we came up with inevitably led us to adopt one or more new beliefs.

Three Shitty Beliefs

1. **I am unlovable.** This includes "I am not _____ enough." As children, we might fill in the blank with words like smart, thin, athletic, old, pretty, tall, or fun. We felt incompetent and insecure, which made us self-conscious, even about doing the things we enjoyed. We stopped trying new things. We felt inferior and ashamed. We avoided all kinds of risks, like putting our hand up in class or taking on leadership roles or voicing an opinion.

2. **My needs are not important.** This translates into feeling unworthy. We may have thought we were fundamentally flawed, that something was really wrong with us. We attracted and befriended people who treated us poorly, because that's what we believed we deserved. In fact, we came to expect it. Some of us even felt like we were a burden, so we made ourselves small in our desire to make life easier for the people we loved. We didn't express our needs, let alone anything we wanted. We likely developed a fear of rejection. If we believed we had little value as a person, self-sabotaging behaviors may have started, and pleasing other people became essential.

3. **The world is unsafe.** We felt helpless and vulnerable. Trusting other people was not in our best interest. We knew about

abandonment. With heightened awareness, we were wary of certain situations and often afraid. Our need for protection and control was paramount. We did all we could to protect ourselves and took on the responsibility to protect the people we loved. We learned the techniques of avoidance and denial. We believed in worst-case scenarios and set about to control our environments with obsessive-compulsive behaviors.

These three fundamental and very shitty beliefs were a result of the way we figured out meanings about whatever it was that had an adverse effect on us. It doesn't matter that our thought process was skewed by our very young and still-developing brains. We didn't know any better. Without the benefit of life experience, it's unreasonable to expect that any child could do better. Most of our issues as adults can be traced back to meanings we came up with as children that led to some version of one or more of these beliefs because, after we made up a meaning and a story, we added some coping mechanisms to go along with them. We had to.

The meanings we invented resulted in shitty beliefs.

Coping Mechanisms

When something awful happened to us as a child, we became afraid of it happening again. How could we not? Our quest when we're young is to learn how the world works and because we had an adverse childhood experience, that quest now included finding a means to protect ourselves. We had to ferret out some way to prevent whatever happened to us from happening again. Or, at the very least, a way to comfort ourselves when the fear, or the pain, was too much. Our new beliefs played a critical role in the ways we coped. If our new coping mechanisms were not conscious and deliberate, they manifested by default, subconsciously.

Here are some examples of how the three shitty beliefs caused us to cope:

We had boundary issues.

We avoided relationships and intimacy.

We withdrew.

We had a poor self-image.

We numbed ourselves.

We had issues with trust.

We blamed ourselves.

We lashed out.

We rescued others.

We stopped caring.

We wet the bed.

We became people-pleasers.

We were afraid.

We were shy.

We were controlling.

We had eating disorders.

We repressed our emotions.

We got sick.

We took huge risks.

We were hypervigilant.

We were cranky.

We had trouble sleeping and concentrating.

We repressed bad memories.

We had obsessive-compulsive disorder, OCD, and
post-traumatic stress disorder, PTSD.

We stuffed our feelings down.

We were promiscuous.

We hurt ourselves.

Adapting to Our Circumstances

Children are smart. They can be very creative in finding ways to protect themselves. As kids, we continued to have relationships with friends
and family, but we began to exercise caution about letting people in. We
continued to participate in the world, but we stopped taking risks. We
learned to mitigate the damage and disappointment before it occurred.
We continued to grow and evolve, but we kept the unique and true
aspects of who we really were hidden under very tight wraps to avoid
ridicule and rejection. We did whatever we had to in order to feel safe.

And we were often completely unaware of what we were doing.
Our still-developing brains (and our inner dialogue) convinced us to
do everything in our power to protect ourselves from further hurt. We
strived to protect our bodies, our environment, and our hearts.

Our quest to protect ourselves
resulted in coping mechanisms.

I'm living proof of how damage done to the heart and mind of a
child lingers well into adulthood. Over the years, I'd heard from several
therapists that everyone's troubles start in childhood. I just didn't give
it any credence. Until I had to. Until the people at The Place gave me
no choice but to see it.

It is possible, with therapy or outstanding adult affection and guidance, that kids can work through and overcome these beliefs before they adopt maladaptive behaviors. Most of us, though, carry on with our childhood coping mechanisms and ultimately drag those perspectives into our adult lives.

Lynda's disappearance, the unintentional parental neglect, and the other shit that happened, well . . . it changed me. How could it not? The night of the wailing I became aware that the world was unsafe. With the overwhelming crisis at hand, I quickly got wise to the fact that my needs were no longer important. And the shitstorm over the next five years confirmed in my mind that I was unlovable and unworthy. That's all there was to it.

Like you and everyone else, I did the best I could. I cowered behind my parents' legs and stopped talking to people. Unsure of myself, I struggled to make simple decisions. I did and said whatever it took to get along and not rock the boat, because inadvertently, I'd become responsible for other people's happiness. More than anything, I was a scaredy cat of epic proportions—afraid of being snatched, of being difficult, of saying the wrong thing, of taking up people's valuable time, of disappointing anyone, of what might happen next, of what people thought of me, and, well, you get the picture. It wasn't pretty. I was especially afraid to speak up for myself. On top of it all, I believed the voice in my head that said it was my job to protect everyone I loved and to ensure their happiness.

So, I took matters into my own hands. Literally. It became easier and safer to do everything myself and not rely on anyone for anything. Newspapers and TV news gave me anxiety. Creating a blissful bubble for myself, I read books and started pulling my hair out at the back of my neck. The pain of the tug on my skin became a soothing comfort that I craved, and before long, it was a constant and unconscious habit that continues to this day.

When we are forced to recognize our made-up stories and look objectively at our responsive behaviors, the false foundation upon which they were built is revealed, and we're able to see their futility.

Fear is always the main culprit. Nothing else can cause us to lose our way so profoundly.

Fear is always the main culprit. Nothing else can
cause us to lose our way so profoundly.

CHAPTER 3

Childhood Fears

We were not born to listen to fear;
we were taught to listen to it.

—James Van Praagh

I 'm told that a few days after my Aunt Lynda's disappearance, my parents sat me down to tell me that she was gone and that they didn't know where or why or when she might come back. They had no answers or explanations for themselves, let alone for me. The fear I sensed that night never left me. The way I figured it, no girls were safe. We were all at risk of being taken. And you never knew if or when it was going to be you.

We weren't born with fear. We learned it. Fears were instilled indirectly by our interpretation of an event. By the voices in our head. The unique things we became afraid of sprouted from the stories we made up and the meanings we concocted with our young brains rather than from the actual event itself.

> The unique things we became afraid of sprouted from
> the stories we made up and the meanings we concocted.

We also learned fears directly from people we trusted. They told us explicitly what we should be afraid of. This was all about them, not us, but as children, we couldn't see that.

Childhood fears are not created equal. They're judged and categorized. We learned that some fears were acceptable and some were not—generally, the more common the fear, the more rational it was deemed. Some fears were dictated by our culture or our religion. The criteria were unique for each of us as our fears were evaluated by our parents, siblings, teachers, and playmates. If our fears were considered irrational, we suffered even more as shame was added. If our fears were judged to be acceptable, they were reinforced and often became worse. Either way, we internalized the verdict. Fear judging is a lose–lose scenario.

Growing up, my mother was extremely dominant. Her intentions were good. Her mission became that of keeping me safe and alive which, in her mind, required more effort than most mothers. To that end, she developed and enforced a list of special rules.

I wasn't allowed to go anywhere after dark. Not walking, not with friends, not by bus, and especially not alone. There were no exceptions. Ever. Because, just in case I ever came close to forgetting (which I tried really hard to do), my mother would remind me regularly, that terrible men grab girls and kill them. There were times I wanted to scream, "Ya, Mom. I know. I know. I KNOW!"

Winters in Canada bring darkness at 4:30 p.m. As a high school student, this meant that all after-school activities were off the table. Without prearranged, Mom-approved transportation, participation in sports or clubs or hanging out anywhere after school was not allowed.

Even going to a friend's house was out of the question. The rule was that I must be safely ensconced in our house before it was dark. To me, this was ludicrous. Especially because my eleven-year-old brother didn't have these special rules. He was a boy. Boys were not at risk.

So.

Not.

Fair.

A voice in my own head confirmed that the risks were indeed real, which kept me on my toes. It forced me to admit that my mom did have a point, and by the same token, it reenforced the fear. Imperative that I faithfully possess an *uber* sense of my personal surroundings, it became second nature for me to gauge the pace and distance of any footsteps behind me, to notice and commit to memory the location of the nearest phone booth, exit stairs, security desk, and human who might save me. A bowl of quarters, free for the taking, sat on the kitchen counter as insurance for my ability to make an emergency phone call. Obviously, I took self-defense lessons. My mother is nothing if not thorough. I hated them. I think my mother conducted this safety training with the maternal inkling that she wouldn't be able to control me forever. In what I can assume was an attempt to balance things out, I also received instruction in female deportment—things like posture, manners, and etiquette—which seemed extremely contradictory, because, for the life of me, I couldn't see how these skills would be any help at all if I ever got snatched.

Throughout my teenage years, I found evidence everywhere, and it mounted up. Looking over my shoulder to see a man on the sidewalk catching up behind me, prompted me to think things like: *See, I knew it! Time to cross the street and pick up the pace. Good thing you were paying attention, Liz!*

The transition from childhood to adulthood is a challenging and awkward stage on so many fronts. Physical developments and emotional shifts send us into a tizzy. The last thing on our minds is any concern about the fact that we're still using our childhood thought processes, rationales, and meanings to figure out all the new stuff that's happening. These are also the years where we're striving for a unique identity and sometimes taking risks. It's unfortunate that our childhood coping mechanisms are still driving the bus.

Children who experience emotional volatility learn to be hypervigilant emotionally. When our needs are not met, we learn that it's better not to rely on anyone, and we typically have problems establishing boundaries. When we're subjected to emotional abuse, we have difficulty identifying boundary violations. And if we endured verbal abuse, we grow up with very low self-worth.

CHAPTER 4

You Did the Best You Could

For in every adult there dwells the child that was,
and in every child there lies the adult that will be.

—*John Connolly*, The Book of Lost Things

While writing this book and reflecting on my childhood, I spent some time talking with my eighty-three-year-old dad. Turns out he's blocked a lot of the Lynda years out of his memory too. My father loves me without reservation. To the moon and back, as they say. There's nothing in the world he wouldn't do for me if it was within his power.

When we talked about the five years that Lynda was missing, he said, "Yeah . . . there were more than a few times when we were really worried about you, and your mother and I did talk about it. But there was so much else happening that demanded our resources. It was a crisis. We just figured that, because you were so young, you'd be okay." My brother, only a toddler at the time, got even less consideration.

My parents assumed I'd get over Lynda's disappearance. They thought they sheltered me sufficiently. After all, I was just a kid. Now, there are a couple ways I could interpret that. I could think my parents were idiots. Or naïve. Or that they didn't care about me. The truth is, it's a natural and often subconscious tendency for all parents to do unto their children as their parents did unto them. It's a chain that's hard to break.

The Blame Game

An obvious choice for our childhood dilemmas is to blame our parents. After all, they were the adults. Legally responsible for us, they surely had control over everything that happened in our childhoods. And, well, if they didn't, they should have. Especially where it concerned their precious children. Right?

We are all at risk of repeating the mistakes of our parents. Today, as a parent myself, I know this. I think of my own efforts as a single mother raising two boys. Easily and without reservation, I'll admit there were times when I also dropped the ball. Lots of times. And my boys know it. I can also now see there were a few occasions where I acted just like my mother. That one hurts to admit, but the shoe fits.

Whether parenthood status arrives as planned or unplanned, easily or after considerable time or expense, the responsibilities are ominous. I believe the majority of parents take their role very seriously. Everyone who is one knows it's one of the toughest jobs in the world. It's also one of the most rewarding.

Blame is a concept that seems to float in the air, all by itself. As kids, we didn't even have to be asked a question. All it took was a *look* from an adult or an older sibling and we started spouting things like, "What?!" or "Wasn't me!" or "I didn't do it!" Heads would swing wildly back and forth meeting the eyes of everyone around and then fingers got pointed. It never ended well when fingers got pointed.

For my entire life, I witnessed my father walk away from any household conflict. He had to do this often, because my mother generated more than her fair share of strife in her quest to control us and the world. Every single time, he acquiesced. It was difficult for me to watch. To myself, I judged his response to these altercations as a weakness of character. I criticized him for "burying his head in the sand" all the time. I loved and accepted him, but I thought he really should learn how stand up for himself more. Fifty years later, I can see the irony of my judgment. Back then, I had no idea how to stand up for myself. In fact, standing up for myself is something that I'm still learning how to do.

Recently, my dad and I had a conversation that changed everything. I was aware that his father was a bad drinker, but I had no idea that my grandfather was physically abusive to his wife. Nor did I know that my father, as a young boy, witnessed and heard this abuse regularly. Sadly, in the 1940s, domestic abuse was acceptable if it was kept indoors. My judgment of how my dad handled the friction generated by my mother took a 180-degree turn. With this new information, I viewed all of his nonactions as the most formidable strength of character and the most valuable gift a father could give his children. My gratitude is immeasurable. He broke the chain.

My dad wasn't alone in his belief that young children are totally resilient to trauma. It's a systemic problem that, only in recent years, is coming to the forefront of therapy and improving with new research. Dr. Bruce D. Perry explains in his book *What Happened to You?* that "people indulge in wishful thinking that a child could experience traumatic stress and somehow, magically be unaffected." His studies confirm that's not the way it works. Our brains are malleable and continue to adapt and change as a result of our experiences. Children's brains are still developing, which makes them even less resilient to trauma, not more.[1]

What else could we blame? Society? God? The school system? Automobile manufacturers? The universe? Whatever our trauma was, there's someone or something that could be blamed. Blame is always available if that's what we're looking for. Sometimes terrible things happen to good people. This is sad but true.

My mother was pregnant when Lynda disappeared.

As the months went by, everyone dealt with their grief and their imaginations in their own way. Brooding about all the possible horrific scenarios of what happened, or worse, what was still happening, to Lynda was inevitable for all of us, but my nana's mind was cruel. Her breakdown affected us immensely. She was the matriarch, the glue of our clan, and it was like she'd been hypnotized by a monster. Grief-driven psychosis caused her to completely shut down.

As my grandfather, whom I had dubbed "Bampa," tended to his wife, my mother filled in to manage the crisis. She did the best she could, but there was a big gap. Multiple search efforts were organized, meetings held with the Ontario Provincial Police (OPP), private detectives were hired, legalities to offer a reward sorted out, endless (mostly crackpot) calls were vetted, contact lists of Lynda's friends and associates were compiled, the validity of psychics confirmed, and communication updates were coordinated for everyone involved. It was a high-stakes responsibility. The stress took a tremendous mental and physical toll on my mother.

At five months pregnant, she went into labor. It was 1968, and the best they could do was give her morphine to stop the contractions. And it worked. Until she went into labor again a few days later. These cycles of labor and morphine continued for weeks, until one day the doctor explained that they could not go on. Any more morphine would render my mom an addict and cause irreparable harm to the baby.

On pins and needles, we waited and hoped for nothing to happen. A few days later my mother went into labor one last time, and my sister Mary-Anne was born weighing about two pounds. My brother and I were not allowed to visit them. Instead, my dad took us every day to the lawn outside the hospital where we would stand, the three of us holding hands, and look up to see our mom waving at us from the window.

My sister lived for five days. Then we buried her. And then my mother completely checked out from parenting.

The days and weeks went on and I somehow knew that until this situation got resolved, until my Aunt Lynda was found, anything I needed was irrelevant. I was afraid to ask. Moreover, it felt selfish and indulgent of me to think that anything at all, particularly me and my brother, were more important than finding Lynda.

It's Not Your Fault

As children, we often blame ourselves for what happened to us. Naively, we believe that we could've changed or prevented something if only we'd acted differently. Most children suppose they are somehow to blame, or are at least partially responsible, for their parents' divorce. Thankfully, this concept is understood, and the misconceptions and associated trauma can be avoided if the divorce is handled with this consideration in mind.

We blame others to give ourselves a free pass. We blame ourselves to justify our helplessness. Eventually, though, we learn that blame is an illusion. Blaming is just another story that we make up to figure things out.

Blaming is just another story that we make up to figure things out.

Sooner or later, everyone who plays the blame game loses. Yet, we continue to play. I blamed my mother for most of my life. I blamed other people, too, for all kinds of things. Only in hindsight can I see the extent to which it impacted my happiness. Not only is it unfair to blame our parents, but it also doesn't serve us. They were doing the best they could too.

We can't change what happened. Through no fault of our own, we became inadvertent victims of our childhoods. That's how we ended up in Victimtown.

Through no fault of our own, we became
inadvertent victims of our childhoods.

PART 2

Victimtown

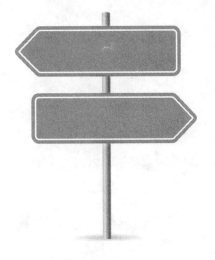

CHAPTER 5

Welcome to Victimtown

Not till we are lost . . .
do we begin to find ourselves.
—*Henry David Thoreau*

W e all try different things to feel better. Sometimes these things help a little bit or work for a little while. But a lot of the things we try fall short of our expectations. The quick fix, the easy answer they all promise is almost always unachievable. We continue to yearn. That's where I was. After all my work at The Place, I was still yearning . . . for the voice in my head to F off, for the drama to stop, to figure out what I'm meant to do, to just . . . to just feel happy. Was this too much to ask? The Place made doing all the right things for my mental health fairly easy while I was there, but integrating all the right things into my real world was another story altogether.

The Yearnings

A yearning is what happens when we're unhappy for too long. It's like a seed inside us—a seed that's begging to sprout and grow. It's undeniable. It's unstoppable. It's innate. I know now that a yearning often arrives as a defense player against our feelings of despair and pain. And that's a good thing. A yearning is not a want; it's not something we choose or can control. It's our heart voice wanting to be heard. A yearning is an awakening.

When a yearning arrives, it's usually a need for one of four sentiments: peace, love, freedom, or joy. I know this is another corny statement, but the truth is, when we really think about it, all the things we want fall into one of those categories. Once a yearning reaches the point of no return, we'll have no solace until we achieve whatever it is we yearn for.

What do you yearn for in the quiet of the night?

To love yourself?

To be in a loving relationship?

To be happy?

For something unwanted to end?

To feel fulfilled or find your purpose?

I yearned for all those things.

I'd been home from The Place for about three months when the shitty voice in my head got loud again and the familiar sense of doom returned. I began to question myself, to worry, to fear. And cry. Like, a lot. I was a bit pissed off about it too. I mean, considering the time and money and the massive emotional undertaking, I thought for sure The Place would fix everything, for now and forever, which I suppose wasn't really fair. Or realistic. It was disappointing AF.

One night, as I lay in bed trying to fall asleep, I began once again to think that my demise was the only solution.

How is it possible, after all the work I've done, to be feeling like this again? I'm too tired to deal with this anymore. I just can't.

At four o'clock in the morning, I woke up with my adrenaline pumping. I was furious and ready for a fight.

Weird. Why am I so mad?

Tidbits of my dream began to come through, and I was met with the most startling revelation. And it wasn't a good one.

Are you kidding me? No effing way. This can't be true. Not me. Not now. The world can go suck it.

I pulled the covers over my head, but it was impossible to fall back asleep. The voices in my head were in a harsh battle that I couldn't control, let alone stop. I tossed and turned, and at five o'clock, I finally surrendered. I got up. And puked.

I was a victim. The concept hit me hard. And that was only the first part. It wasn't just that I was a victim, it was that I'd been living with a victim mentality my entire life!

How could I have been so blind?

And the punch to finish me off was that I continued to rely on the coping mechanisms that I adopted as a kid. All that armor was starting to grow heavy.

How did I not feel the weight of it all? Why was I was holding on tightly to this righteousness? Was I that naïve and obtuse? Why didn't they just tell me this at The Place?

My victimhood had become so much a part of who I was that I didn't even notice it was there, probably because it had been there since I was six years old.

Mad as hell, I got up and started journaling (a new habit carried over from The Place). As my words hit the pages, new insights emerged. My problems only partly stemmed from my childhood. The real issue, all my current problems, were not because of what happened to me but because of how tightly I was holding on to the stories I made up to explain it all.

My strategy for healing, or finishing my healing, needed a creative approach. I was completely covered with armor and could feel the weight of it on my heart. It was very, very heavy. The work I'd done so far had helped. I mean, I did shed a decent amount of armor at The Place. But I also held on to some. Just in case. To cover the vital parts, ya know?

There it was. This new knowledge did not sit well with me. Not at all. I may have been collateral damage, but the real victim was Lynda, not me.

Then something surprising happened—a reassuring voice showed up, and I heard it loudly. I felt comforted by what it had to say, so I decided to call it my heart voice.

This information is a gift. If you view it like that, everything will be okay. You can become an anti-victim.

That message felt true. Even though it would be hard, peeling the armor away from my heart, layer by layer, was the only answer. A single requirement that sounded straightforward, but when it comes to matters of the heart, not much is ever straightforward. And I wasn't naïve about the self-help journey; my time at The Place taught me that. There was only one person with the capacity to get this job done. Me. I thought objectively about everything I learned at The Place, and the truth is, they never promised me a quick and easy fix. That was just wishful thinking on my part. What they did promise was to teach me the tools to do it for myself.

There's only one person with the
capacity to get this job done. YOU.

Now, don't go get in a tizzy and throw this book away yet. Hear me out. I realize that being called a victim doesn't feel very nice. When I hear the word victim, the first thing that comes to mind is someone who's had something terrible done to them through absolutely no fault of their own. For many people, the word victim brings up feelings of shame. It's not an honorable label. Or is it?

All Victims Are Not Created Equal

We often think of a victim as a person harmed, injured, or killed as a result of a crime, accident, or other event. Or maybe someone who was deceived or cheated. Based on that, pretty much every one of us qualifies as a victim at some point in our lives. We can be victims by definition or by default, simply because of what happened to us. We have no control over becoming a victim. And it's not necessarily a bad thing.

If we had any trauma whatsoever in our childhood, we grew up to become a victim of some kind or another. All victims, however, are not created equal. It's possible for people to flow from one victim type to another or to embody a combination of these three types.

1. **The Whiners.** At one end of the spectrum, we have the victims who are whiners and complainers. Nothing in their entire lives is ever their fault. They have a long list of experiences to justify their plight. Nothing ever goes right for them. They have a chip on their shoulder. With their attitude of entitlement, you can sense their negativity just by being in the same room. They expect, and secretly delight in, things going wrong. They feel completely justified in their victimhood. Without reservation, they are proud of it and often brag about it. Having earned their victim status, they always have a story that's just a little bit worse than the one somebody else is telling. Their armor is worn with pride, and they carry the weight without difficulty. Or so it seems. In a large way, it defines their personality.

2. **The Private Victims.** Not all victims are complainers though, nor are they all Negative Nellies. Some of them keep their victimhood private. They're aware of why and how they became

victims, but they don't really want the world to know. On occasion, when they're feeling courageous, they might share vulnerable feelings with people they trust. Secretly though, they view themselves as weak or not good enough. They're embarrassed or, worse, they feel ashamed about some fundamental aspect of themselves or about something that happened. Putting up a good front, they soldier on and don't complain. But they struggle. They feel the effects of the heavy armor on their hearts every day, even though they may be unaware of it. Anxiety and depression are common among this type. On their bad days, they are incapacitated. On their good days, they seek solutions for their unhappiness. Alcohol is consumed more nights than not. They would love nothing more than to feel better, but they lack an actionable plan.

3. **The High-Functioning Victims.** Most of this group have no idea they hold a victim mentality. If they do have an inkling, they dismiss it. Not able or ready to consider victimhood a possibility, it usually takes a huge life-disrupting event for them to figure it out themselves. These victims are extremely high functioning. Making up a very large portion of the population, these folks don't have to try to hide it, because they don't even know they have it. To the outside world, they seem to have their shit together. Their lives appear under control. Yet, they continue to produce unwanted behavior patterns. They find themselves dealing with failed relationships, drama and unfortunate circumstances, and high stress over and over. Questioning their lot in life, they attempt to resign themselves to the way things are. Like the high-functioning alcoholic, these high-functioning victims are managing to hold things together. Under the surface, however, there's a problem. They're not happy. Feelings of unfulfillment are causing the seeds of a yearning to grow. The connection to their childhood traumas has not yet been made.

They're so used to the weight of the armor on their hearts, it doesn't bother them at all. They have no idea it's even there; they can't feel it. Yet. That was me.

The more I kept thinking about my dream and how I woke up covered in armor, the more I started to remember. The town in my dream felt familiar from my time at The Place. As I daydreamed sometimes during group therapy, I thought about these places. The Control Factory sat proudly at the end of the main road. A restaurant called the Guilt & Shame Café bustled with rowdy customers, and the Resentment Parking Lot next door was full. In the distance, beyond the Sorrow Swampland, I could see the entrance for the Denial Trails. The Anger Gas Station had a lineup, and the Ego Arena's marquee advertised an upcoming event. There was hardly anyone in the Meditation Meadow and too many people at Epiphany Hospital.

I live here. I've lived here most of my life.

And then the name came to me. Victimtown.

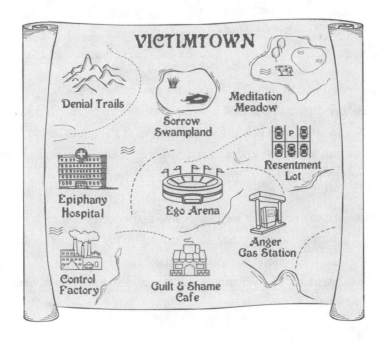

The Population of Victimtown

It's not pleasant to admit you have a victim mentality. Yet, we all do have it at some point in our lives, for our own reasons, about distinct issues, for varying amounts of time. I was six years old when I started to listen to the voices of Victimtown. Like most of us, I had no idea what I was doing. Nor did I recognize the voices in each place for what they really were. They were loud and convincing, and I believed every single thing they said.

Every person on earth shows up in Victimtown at one time or another. Victims of crime, yes, but all the good people who are dealt undeserving blows of any description can also be found here. Victimtown is where we go when we're not quite ready to face the pain. It's an equal-opportunity place for all humans. This includes detectives and perpetrators, too. That's because the people who've caused us pain are in at least as much pain themselves.

Victimtown is where we go when we're not quite ready to face the pain.

It's not a bad thing to land in Victimtown. On the contrary, all the places here can serve our best interests. Naming them has the power to jolt us into awareness of our futile behaviors. It's much easier to figure out our shit when we know exactly where we are. Personal growth abounds in Victimtown. Opportunities for learning and healing reside here. It's essential that we hang out here for a certain amount of time because it's the only way we can evolve and become better humans. Could it be that learning our soul lessons is the purpose of life? I believe this is the reason each of us visits Victimtown.

Fulfillment of our yearnings, however, doesn't happen here. It can't. Nor will we find our purpose. You won't find peace, freedom, or joy in Victimtown. Although love is with us wherever we are, love's not in abundance here, nor does it grow well in this climate. The weather in Victimtown is stormy and dark. The only place where the sun peaks through is over the Meditation Meadow.

I know every place in Victimtown intimately. Without exception. This was my home for most of my life. It's much older than me, though. It's been around forever! The buildings are ancient, but they've stood the test of time. Well maintained, they've been modified over the years, mixing their old charm seamlessly with modern additions. You will most certainly find one or more of these places familiar.

The Ego Arena's irresistible marketing efforts lure us into Victimtown. Entertainment abounds in this massive gathering place. We're all too afraid of missing the show to leave. Voices on a loud-speaker amplify the voice in each of our own minds with a mission to dial up the drama and chaos and instill fear.

The Control Factory is where my mother had a long career, my ex-husband too. And a few ex-boyfriends. Okay, almost all of them. Because I worked there myself most of my life, I didn't meet many people anywhere else. The Boss upholds the three shitty beliefs as core values of this company. I toiled tirelessly to achieve success here.

The Maître D' would show me to the private back room of the Guilt & Shame Café. He'd say, "You are completely inadequate," as he set a bottle of wine on the table for me. I deserved to be there.

With my bullhorn ready in the trunk, I was a champion grudge-holder for a long, long, long time. I still catch myself pulling into the Resentment Parking Lot on occasion. It used to be fun to park there and laugh heartily at people who did me wrong and judge them for all of their inadequacies.

Although I didn't fill up at the Anger Gas Station often, I knew where it was. I used the fuel from time to time and I was also along for the ride on many occasions. The owner would yell, "You don't have to stand for this. Do something!"

Inevitably, I'd end up floating in the Sorrow Swampland . . . listening to a soft voice singing to me that I'd never be able to move on . . . and I'd try not to sink to the bottom . . . but I wondered if I'd find peace there. . . .

Whenever I got tired of bouncing around from one place to the next, I'd head for the Denial Trails. Always such a vibrant and fun place—at least that's what everyone thinks. I've logged so many miles on these trails that my hiking boots are threadbare.

I should also let you know that each of the places in Victimtown has its own voice. You may have heard their messages yourself. All the town voices are violent communicators. They're manipulative and coercive in a very crafty and unstoppable way. At least there is one location of reprieve here: the Meditation Meadow. It's the only quiet place in Victimtown, and it's very special.

I learned there are no rewards for overstaying your welcome, only suffering. Whether you've just arrived or have been here for years, you'll find that birds of a feather most definitely flock together in each of the places found here.

There are unlimited routes both into and out of Victimtown, some are just harder to see or to navigate than others. A lot of us will know how we got here, but more people than you'd think just wake up one day (or one night) completely taken aback to realize they're living in Victimtown.

But here's the thing: This is a good realization because it's really, really hard to move forward or make a change without first knowing exactly where we are. Only by accepting the complete reality of our situation—every scary aspect of ourselves, even, perhaps especially, the ugly truth—will we be equipped to move on. Acceptance is only for the present moment, and we don't have to like it. Frequently, if we're honest, the present moment can suck. We don't need to feel good about it, but if we continue to deceive ourselves about where we are and what we're doing, we'll become stuck in Victimtown. And although it's okay to visit for a short time, big problems arise and unhappiness settles in when we hang out in Victimtown too long.

On top of that, the longer we stay, the harder it can be to leave. And take it from me—it's not always easy to sort out the voices in our head. It's a good thing, though, when we start to feel confused. That means the seeds of a yearning are beginning to sprout. When we start to wonder where to go or what to do, when we start to question if we're on the right path, that's our heart voice begging to be heard.

There's always a way out. Once we learn whatever lesson we need to learn in Victimtown, new paths are revealed. Paths that lead to Freedomville. We learn our lessons by the act of feeling. There's no other way. It can be hard and scary to leave some of these places, particularly when we're deeply ensconced, but it's harder and more terrifying to stay once you know where you are. I think you'll find at least one place in Victimtown familiar. In fact, I guarantee it.

Victimtown can be the place of our demise. Or the place of our healing. We all get to choose.

Victimtown can be the place of our demise. Or the place of our healing. We all get to choose.

Once we know something, we can't unknow it. New insights can bring a sense of relief, especially when the new knowledge surrounds a struggle. You can call it horse sense if you want, but this new insight was my fresh approach. Even without a solid plan and even before I took the first step, I felt reassured. I was newly armed with an arsenal of strategies that I learned at The Place. It was time to try them out. Realizing I was living in Victimtown was the best thing that ever happened to me. For real.

It arrived 19,082 days after Lynda went missing.

CHAPTER 6

The Ego Arena

The first principle is that you must not fool
yourself, and you are the easiest person to fool.
—*Richard Feynman*

My mom is the oldest of five with three boys in the middle between her and her little sister. They're a close and loving family, raised in the 1950s in a safe suburban town in southern Ontario, Canada. When my aunt disappeared, the three oldest siblings were already married, living on their own, and working full time. The younger two, Bobby and Lynda, were in their second and first years, respectively, at nearby universities.

The phone call came in mid-November from one of Lynda's roommates: "She hasn't been home for two days, and we haven't heard from her. Nobody knows where she is." It was something none of us were prepared for.

Last seen shortly after taking a midterm exam, Lynda was a varsity athlete and a decent student. She was kind and very well liked. And she was beautiful. At six years old, all I knew was that she was my favorite aunt and sleepovers with her were the best thing ever.

I was startled awake from a deep sleep by a strange sound. At first, I thought I was dreaming, but when I opened my eyes, I could still hear the sound. It was like nothing I'd ever heard before, and I had no idea where it was coming from. It started out softly, but now it elevated to pitches and wails that sent shivers down my spine. It reminded me of *Mutual of Omaha's Wild Kingdom,* because it sounded like an animal. A very large, dying animal. It was guttural. I clamped my small hands over my ears. Whatever was making that sound was in intense pain. But the worst part was, it was in my house!

My imagination ran wild. My bedroom door was open a few inches. Looking into the hallway from the safety of my bed, I could see that the door to my parents' bedroom was closed. I wanted to know for sure where the sound was coming from, but I was afraid to listen harder.

Please make it stop. Please. Make it stop.

One finger at a time, I unclamped my hands from my ears. I lay there exposed for a nanosecond, before I quickly covered my eyes. As my senses recalibrated, I realized the cries were indeed coming from my parents' bedroom. Certain that someone was dying, I had the feeling it might be my mother. I slid deeper under the covers, but the sounds found me there, and I started to cry.

Who will look after me if my mommy dies? What could be doing this to her? Where is my daddy? What if it comes to get me next? Am I going to die too?

As I lay hidden in my bed, I remembered my little brother in his room at the far end of the hall. He was barely two years old.

Can he hear this too? Is he crying all alone in his crib?

I wanted to go see him, to comfort him, but I couldn't move. So, I waited. And I wished with all my might for the world to be silent. But the quiet didn't arrive. And when the wailing got even louder, my worry for my baby brother escalated and I couldn't wait any longer for my wishing to work. I took a deep breath and stepped onto the bare floor. With one thumb in my mouth and the other hand over my ear, I began to tiptoe very, very slowly down the hall as quiet as a mouse. Peeking around the corner into his room, I saw that he was wide awake.

Standing up in his crib, he had his chubby little fingers curled tightly around the top railing. He looked confused. He was just standing there, staring at nothing, but at least he wasn't crying. I moved closer and he saw me. He smiled. The wailing wasn't as loud in his room, and I didn't want to be alone, so I climbed into his crib. One by one, I pried his fingers off the railing. He plopped down on his bum, and we curled up together. The lump in my stomach was so big that it filled my throat and almost choked me.

What's going to happen to us now?

The hub of Victimtown, the gathering place for all, is the Ego Arena at the center of town. Voices on a loudspeaker amplify the voice in each of our minds—ego voices. Talking over each other, the voices are incessant and loud to the point of being overbearing. Our amped-up ego voices are in charge of the arena. Their singular mission is to instill FEAR. Each takes cues from another. Ego voices learn and evolve by listening to the others on the loudspeaker. They say the strangest things to convince us not to leave. Each voice is an instigator with a mission to incite and control us. It meddles in every aspect of our lives, because it's desperate to keep us in the arena where it can be heard.

We show up here to be entertained and also to attract attention to ourselves. Competition is fierce for the good seats. Nobody really likes it here, but nobody wants to leave either. With florescent lighting and an absence of windows, the recirculated air is stale. Wall-to-wall people are out for themselves, steadfastly shoving their way toward the better seats. We have little regard for others in our quest to attain a private box. Nobody stops to help anybody else. Yet, nobody wants anybody else to leave.

You can forget about a better view. Box seats are for the elite, and there are very few available. It's common knowledge that these seats are reserved for the people who are the richest and the most beautiful. They have the biggest house, the best careers, the best bodies, the most accomplished children, couture fashion, the highest education, revered status, and engaging personalities.

If we enjoy a reasonably good seat in this arena, we feel lucky because we believe there aren't enough good seats for everyone. At the same time, we think we're better and more deserving than the folks in the cheap seats. If we can see the worst section, we feel sorry for them. We should be grateful to be where we are, but deep down, we're not happy. The voices convince us that all of our problems will disappear if and when we get box seats.

Anyone who's achieved box seats feels special and entitled. Some people relish the segregation and only invite guests into their box to impress them with their status. As we view other seats from our box, our superiority confirms our success.

And if we have a shitty seat, well, we're bitter and scheming about the unfairness of it all. What are we even doing here? Everyone compares themselves to everyone else. Our worth in the arena is measured by things, with money at the top of the list.

A clue that we're in the Ego Arena is when we think things like, *I'll be happy when* _____ *happens.* We can all fill in the blank. When I'm thinner, I get a new car, buy a bigger house, my kid stops getting in trouble, my brother moves away, my brother moves closer, I win the lottery. The list is endless. We believe that something needs to *happen* in order to be happy.

There's lots of drama in the Ego Arena. We pick arguments daily. Fanatical in our mission to be right (the cost of which is irrelevant), we set out to force our will on the world. We understand there are only so many good seats available. If we don't grab one for ourselves and defend it, someone will take it away from us. The competition is fierce and dirty.

Gossip is a favorite pastime in the Ego Arena. We rarely address our issues with people directly. Instead, we stand around and talk about them with everyone else. We discuss their shortcomings, their failures, their inabilities, their negative qualities, and their mistakes. Not only is gossiping fun, but it also makes us feel infinitely better about ourselves because judging others provides relief.

With an uncanny ability to take total advantage of our most vulnerable bits, the voice in the arena pinpoints and highlights all of our weaknesses. Using words alone, it can control and destroy us. The ultimate trickster, the voice pretends to be us. It humiliates us and makes us take everything personally. Our ego voice can justify anything.

A favorite activity of the ego voice is to stir up obsessive, ruminating thoughts, which can really get us going. Anxiety is its main goal, as it feeds on our stress hormones. This voice complains about everything. Overusing the word *should,* it spews a never-ending stream of instructions.

The ego voice says things like, "You're not smart enough," "You should expect bad things to happen," and "You should just suck it up."

These loudspeaker voices reinforce any of the three shitty beliefs we picked up in childhood. Regardless, we learn to feel at home in this arena and we settle in.

As terrible as the arena sounds, we're all naturally drawn to the arena by some invisible force. Many people choose to spend much of their time here. They thrive in this environment and hear nothing but the voices on the loudspeaker. Some of us, however, get sick of listening to this shit when we feel a yearning seed starting to grow inside us. When this happens, we begin to look for a way out.

EMDR

I likened the people at The Place to diggers. They were master excavators. They were the emotional counterpart to the massage therapist who knows exactly where to find that tiny little muscle with a knot in it that you didn't even know existed and that hurt like hell when they pressed their thumb into it. Yowza! Likewise, my psychotherapist at The Place found the memory I was holding onto about the wailing in no time. Her treatment plan for this little number was EMDR, which stands for Eye Movement Desensitization and Reprocessing.

Say whaaaattttt??

The memory of my mom wailing was still very traumatic for me. I relived the fear and panic every time I thought about it, let alone talked about it. Fifty years later, the feelings had not yet disintegrated like I'd hoped, and I would still become paralyzed with fear and anxiety. And if wine was involved, I would blubber. So, obviously, I tried to avoid doing that. Instead, I pushed that sucker down and locked it up tight.

You might be wondering, what exactly is EMDR? EMDR is a fairly new, nontraditional type of psychotherapy.[1] It's becoming more popular because of its effectiveness. EMDR is a means to help our brains make new pathways so they can resolve unprocessed traumatic memories. I know. It sounded kinda weird to me too at first. I was skeptical, but willing to give it a go.

After two sessions of foundational work and setup to keep me safe, my appointment had arrived to do the EMDR thingy.

"Okay. Let's get started," my therapist said. "I want you to look forward at me and keep your head still. I'm going to move my finger back and forth, and I want you to follow it only with your eyes. After you get the hang of it, I'm going to ask you to recall the event that night and walk me through everything that happened, but you can't stop following my finger with your eyes."

Shit. This sounds complicated.

"Okay, I'll try."

Mustering every ounce of concentration, I began to follow her finger, doing the eye movement. Her finger was moving fast—too fast! Instinctively, my head began to help my eyeballs keep up with this rapid back and forth. I'm not a total dork. I mean, it wasn't an exorcist maneuver or anything. Just a subtle two-inches-to-the-left-then-two-inches-to-the-right kind of movement that I thought might be okay.

"Umm. Please try to keep your head still and just move your eyes," she said.

I concentrated harder. It looked like I was getting it, so she moved to the next phase.

"Tell me what happened that night," she said.

So, I did. But as soon as I started talking, my head began moving again. My brain completely balked at doing those two things at once. When I thought about the memory, my eyes stopped following her finger. Many months later, when I got diagnosed with attention deficit disorder (yup, at the age of fifty-nine), this made so much more sense. At any rate, there was another option to achieve the same result.

EMDR can also be done by tapping. Sitting in a chair, I crossed my arms so that, with my hands flat, my fingers were resting on my opposite shoulders. Moving only my wrists, I began to simultaneously tap my shoulders with both hands. As I tapped quickly, it didn't take long for me to get into a *zone,* and the repetitious movements allowed my brain to think about the memory.

I closed my eyes and continued tapping my shoulders. As I relived the sounds I heard and my thoughts about everything that happened that night, tears streamed down my face and my heart pounded. I felt the panic, the fear, and the pain with more intensity than ever.

"Don't stop tapping. Keep your eyes closed." My therapist gently pushed for more details and new revelations. She also asked me to focus on my body's response—particularly what emotions and feelings I was noticing and where in my body I felt them.

Previously, my memory ended with me getting out of bed and walking toward my bedroom door.

"It's okay. You can leave your bedroom. Where do you go?"

For the first time, I remembered tiptoeing down the hallway into my brother's room. When I relived seeing him standing in his crib, I started sobbing uncontrollably. I kept tapping and she kept reassuring me that I was safe. She led the way for me to process all the feelings that I'd ignored or denied about that night. Feeling my feelings, I came to learn, is like kryptonite for the Victimtown voices that try to keep me trapped inside my old memories.

At the end of our EMDR session, I visualized placing this memory into my imaginary box outside the window in the room we were in. Established in a previous therapy session, this was a *holding box* for issues I was working on so I didn't continue to keep them buried inside myself. I could retrieve them as required in therapy sessions.

It was all kind of surreal. I stopped tapping at last and opened my eyes. Amazed that I remembered more about the night we learned my aunt was missing, I said, "Is that really what happened, or did I make that up?"

"That's what really happened," she said. "Your brain just unlocked the information."

"Huh," was all I could get out. I was completely spent, both physically and emotionally, but the session had a final component. She asked me to recount the events of that scary night one more time, out loud, which I did. It was the strangest thing. I could tell the story, a longer version now, without the fear or the panic. I still felt sad, but the story was softened somehow. It was manageable. And I felt lighter.

She explained that my brain had now formed new, safer connections with the images, thoughts, and emotions from that memory. These new connections allowed my brain to process and resolve it. The total time for the EMDR session was just less than two hours. Not all traumatic memories can be reprogrammed in one session. Another guest at The Place had debilitating PTSD from multiple and continuous traumatic events. Although her EMDR therapy was ongoing, she was making good progress too.

Your Heart Voice

The good news is this: The shitty voice on the loudspeaker in the Ego Arena isn't the only one there. There's a softer voice as well. It's the one that responds when the ego voice speaks. Yet both voices are in our heads. If one voice is talking *to* us, then that voice can't *be* us. And if that voice is *not* us, then what *is* that voice? And which one is our *true voice*?

Our true voice, our essence, is the one we were all born with. It's inside every one of us, waiting patiently to be heard. I call it our *heart voice*. Our heart voice honors our intrinsic human value. Our heart voice has great power. Our heart voice operates the retractable roof of this arena and lets some sunshine in. When the light hits the arena, we can truly see where we are. Let's not be fooled. The people, the structure—everything—becomes apparent with the light. We become conscious and aware.

> Our true voice, our essence, is the one we were all born with—our *heart voice*.

We all have two voices in our heads. Each place in Victimtown has a different voice that says different things. But everything any of the town voices have to say is shit. In the Ego Arena, the loudspeaker is obnoxious and blaring and hard to tune out. It's our enemy. And what do they say about enemies? Keep your friends close and your enemies closer.

The Gifts Found in the Ego Arena

The Ego Arena exists to teach us that we possess a heart voice. When we're sick and tired of listening to the bullshit blasted on the loudspeaker, we'll be willing to explore something better to listen to. Our heart voice will calm us, reassure us, and show us how to leave the arena. When we slow down, tune in, and listen, we can feel our bodies from the inside, and we know the truth of what this voice is telling us. It speaks ever so softly at first, and we might have to strain to hear it. Our heart voice will cheer us on by telling us that we're okay, everything will be alright, and that we already have everything we need.

When we learn how to stay out of the arena, we're not as tempted to visit the other places in Victimtown. It always feels so much better to listen to the messages our heart voice delivers.

We all visit this arena from time to time. Landing here for a brief stay reminds us to be humble. It gives us a chance to practice the concept of intrinsic human value. We come to understand that in no way do our seats determine our worth. Or our happiness. We can become less pretentious. We learn that judgment serves no one. We decipher that competition is an outdated concept.

The Ego Arena can be inspiring, or it can be demoralizing. It depends on which voice we choose to listen to. And the loudspeaker is really, really LOUD. Although the arena is usually the first location we visit in Victimtown, we almost always check out a few other places before we're ready to leave.

CHAPTER 7

The Control Factory

This is a very complicated case, Maude. You know,
a lotta ins, a lotta outs, a lotta what-have-yous.
—*The Dude*, The Big Lebowski *(1998)*

N ot long after my baby sister died, a girl disappeared from the woods right beside my school playground. It happened on the weekend, and she didn't go to my school, but she was the same age as me, and it happened in the same woods that my friends and I played in every day at recess. While my brother and I were still at the dinner table, my parents were talking with each other about this new development. And they remembered something. They said that Marianne Schuett still hadn't been found.

Who was that?

Listening to them, I learned that just last year, ten-year-old Marianne Schuett had gotten into a car when her school let out. She was never seen again. Her school was only nine miles away.

What? It's not just my Aunt Lynda and the girl in the woods?

Another girl got taken last year too?

It sounds hard to believe. But it's true.

After this, my father started walking a group of us neighborhood kids the three blocks to school every morning. With a pitchfork. It completely boggled my mind that we even owned such a thing. I guess it was the only tool in our shed that could be used for protection. The risk of getting snatched just became even more real. All the kids were scared, but nobody was more afraid than me, because I knew firsthand that it didn't just happen to other people.

You'd think I'd remember something as ridiculous as my father holding a pitchfork while walking down the sidewalk, but I don't. That part was told to me by the other kids and also by my dad. What I do remember is being terrified. I was terrified to be alone every single time I left my house. Going to school was non-negotiable. In my classroom, I started looking around.

One, two, three, four . . . there are thirty-six kids here. Whew. That's a lot!

If I can just stay really small. And quiet. And not do anything to stand out . . . if the snatcher shows up here, hopefully he won't see me.

It's not that I wanted anyone else to disappear. I really didn't. That's just how the voice in my head worked back then.

My refusal to leave the safety net of the classroom, however, also meant that I wouldn't even go to the washroom. Not ever. Not even at lunch. Too embarrassed to ask the teacher if a friend could go with me, I didn't want the kids to know I was such a scaredy cat. I was ashamed. And it was a very long day until school let out at 3:45 in the afternoon.

One winter day, when the last bell finally rang, I had to go to the bathroom really, really badly. I don't know why, but nobody was ever around to walk us home. Instead, each of our parents gave us instructions: "Whatever you do, stay together," "Make sure you come straight home," "Don't dilly-dally and don't talk to anyone," and lastly, "Pay attention; keep your wits about you!"

That day, I debated about staying with the group like I was supposed to, but my bladder was about to burst, and they all walked so slowly. We were just a group of kids; we didn't even have a spoon, let alone a pitchfork. The way I figured it, running by myself, as fast as I could the whole way, well, that was my best option.

I happened to be wearing a brand-new outfit. Dark green polyester pants with a seam right down the center of each leg to the coolest bell-bottom flare ever. My plaid top was a perfect match. I was stylin'. The voice in my head, however, was very concerned about something else.

Oh my gosh. I have to go SO bad!! This is NOT good.

Then a different voice showed up.

It'll be okay. Jut run. Run your fastest! And don't look back!

So, I took off at lightning speed. Holding onto the handle of my schoolbag for dear life, I raced down the sidewalk. I couldn't help but look over my shoulder every few steps, and after only two blocks, I could barely breathe. As I rounded the last corner, I could see my house. *Yay!* But it was still more than a block away. Afraid that I was not going to make it, I pretended I was on the track team with a coach on the sidelines yelling at me, "RUN FASTER, LONG!" And I did. Somehow, I found even more energy, and I was able to pick up the pace. But the extra effort expended for that gain in speed, well, let's just say it wasn't the best move. It began to compromise my ability to hold in the pee.

It started with just a few drips. I could feel each one, slowly rolling down the inside of my legs, separately chasing that fateful drop that led the way. I slowed down to a jog, hoping to get a grip, as they say, to stop the flow. But as any girl knows, once that dam breaks, it's damn hard to stop. The pee continued to roll, quickly becoming an unstoppable stream and gaining in velocity, down both legs.

Oh noooo, I hope it doesn't show.

With my shitty luck, it was cold out. Freezing cold. January in Canada cold. And I wished desperately for the safety and privacy of home. The faster I ran, the more I peed.

Ugh . . . my best school clothes are ruined!

It didn't take long for the pee to soak right through the fabric of my green polyester pants, and what followed was like a freakish science experiment. As the warm pee met the frigid winter air, the result was disastrous! Gusts of urine-smelling steam began to rise up around me.

Ewwww . . . yuukkkk . . . what is happennnningggg?

I felt like Pigpen from Charlie Brown, and I started to cry. You'd think that was bad enough, but the science experiment was about to enter phase two. My fancy pants with the pleat down the middle began to get brittle. And then they froze. Solid. I could barely move my legs. Hell was freezing over. My run mutated into a weird, happy-go-lucky, straight-leg-swinging-out-the-sides kind of movement.

I must look like an idiot. Why couldn't I live in Florida?

As my wet skin rubbed and chaffed against the frozen fabric, my legs began to feel like they were on fire, which made no sense at all. I glanced down. There were no flames, but my legs were burning, and to make matters worse, I had frozen tears on my face.

I was very confused.

Ohhh, I can't think about this right now.

It turned out I didn't have to. Because I'd arrived. I'd made it. Back in my warm house, standing there, I looked down at myself. I was melting. My pants were melting.

But I didn't get snatched; not this time anyway.

Otherwise known as just the "factory," the Control Factory is the longest-standing business in Victimtown. It's been passed down from generation to generation. It loses money every year, but it stays open because it has a never-ending supply of people who will work here. For free. I started as a young apprentice with my mom as my manager. Over many years, I put a ton of energy and overtime hours into working here as I moved up the ranks and learned to manage not only other people, but also everything else in the world. I've only recently quit. Truth be told, I think I probably worked here long enough for it to be considered retirement, but with the worst party and no pension.

The people who gravitate to this enterprise are all of us who, at a vulnerable time in our lives, felt subjected to the forces of other people or circumstances out of our control. It's natural for us to respond with a strong pull to control whatever we can. To avoid those nasty, unwanted feelings, especially the pain, we work hard to make everything exactly the way we want it to be. It makes a lot of sense. By listening to the voice of the Boss, we're convinced we can overcome any of the three shitty beliefs by working harder and harder at the factory.

We come to the conclusion that working here, giving it our all, will validate our self-worth, make us lovable, and ensure not only our safety, but also the safety of everyone we love. We learn to depend on our ability to control as much as possible. Certainly, when we are completely in charge, life will be perfect. When the world is exactly the way we need it to be, when everyone does what we want them to do, all of humanity will be happy. Uh-huh. Okay. Sure.

The factory offers an apprenticeship program, which includes temporary employment and lifetime career opportunities at all levels. The Boss tells us we cannot trust ourselves. We must listen to her at all times. She convinces us that she knows how to erase the feeling of being overwhelmed. She knows how to make us happy. And if one job doesn't work out, we can blame someone else. Blaming is not only acceptable; it's expected behavior at the factory. The assignments here can be grueling, requiring a ton of mental energy 24/7. Every. Single. Day. Vacation days? Are you kidding? Our responsibilities are all-consuming, and the tasks are endless. Without exception, our duties are essential. We barely have time to eat, let alone time to look after ourselves or take a break. We believe that working overtime hours to keep constantly busy will help ease, and possibly erase, our sense of helplessness. At least we're not sitting around doing nothing. Or worse, sitting around feeling.

The Work Is Endless

Naturally, our duty here is often for the people we love. Without our hard work, the people we care about wouldn't thrive. Our motivation is self-less. Without a doubt, we know what's best for someone else. Whatever their own ideas are, we've got better ones for them. As parents, the stakes are high. There's a lot of pressure for parents to take on multiple assign-ments at the factory. Everyone knows that one of the hardest jobs here is to ensure that our kids make the right decisions and that they always act appropriately. If we do listen to the opinions of our children (or anyone else), we're ordered by the Boss to set them aside—for their own good, of course. They don't know what they need. We're the only ones who have the necessary credentials and experience to manage them.

When it comes to our partners or friends, the first thing we do after we make our judgment is convince ourselves that they are the ones who need to change. Naturally, we believe it's our responsibility to direct and manage that change. Sometimes, we feel confident; we have a plan. But even if we don't, we'll do whatever it takes to figure it out and make it happen. Whatever they think, feel, or want is not nearly as important as what we know.

We have a job to do. Most of the time we use our skills to help people we care about, but occasionally we work for the demise of people we dislike. Satisfaction is the result when we contribute to an outcome detrimental to someone. After all, the Boss tells us, "They deserved it. So there."

You should know that the Boss at the Control Factory is a tyrant. Her voice on the loudspeaker spills over from the arena into the fac-tory with never-ending jabs:

"When you get them to change, then you'll be happy."

"They shouldn't feel that way."

"You can save them from heartbreak."

Every day, we are tasked to direct, advise, convince, and manage. We only get promoted when we perfect our ability to completely control outcomes. Some people love this work and are very good at it. Others don't like it as much, but they're convinced it's unavoidable. The Boss reiterates our responsibilities and what's expected of us. We think we don't really have a choice. To not work here means we're lazy or we don't care. Little respect is given to anyone who doesn't know how to do at least one factory job. To make matters worse, we're often subjected to the demands of our managers while also striving to do our own jobs.

The Boss says that the way to end our pain is to get people to do what we want. We believe happiness requires ideal circumstances, circumstances that we are somehow responsible for producing. Only by achieving the most ideal outcomes can we feel fulfilled. It's impossible to be happy unless certain things occur.

The factory has three main departments: People, Circumstances, and Events. And we all have our unique affinity to each department. The skills the factory teaches in the People Department, from entry-level positions up to management, range from advice-giving and blaming to gaslighting and guilt-tripping all the way up to threats and abuse.

We use these tactics on other people, but we also use some of them on ourselves. Thankfully, most people work at the entry- and mid-level jobs. There are no labor laws here, and there's certainly no internal affairs division or human resources. Not in Victimtown.

The People Department

This is arguably the largest and most important department in the factory. At times, we work only for ourselves to get ahead and achieve all the things we want. This is supposed to be the easiest job in the factory. Except it's not. We struggle valiantly to not be our own worst enemy.

As an executive at the Control Factory, my husband traveled for work more than he was home. I uncovered his secret life in another state when I was five months pregnant with our second child. Feeling large, tired, and unattractive, I wasn't surprised. He apologized and vowed to embrace monogamy.

A few months after our son was born, he came up with a "great idea." He said, "It's a bit expensive, but totally worth it."

"What is it?" I asked.

"I'm gonna get your boobs fixed."

What? Oh . . . okay. I guess that explains the woman in Duluth.

I didn't mind my small boobs. I mean, sometimes I wished they were a bit bigger, like when the bikini bottoms fit, but the top was too big. But when the stores started selling the pieces separately, I considered the issue solved.

I interpreted his great idea as a statement, a memo of an upcoming project. I never considered it appropriate for me to weigh in. When he asked if I wanted to research doctors, I was surprised. And suspicious. Doubting my skills to perform the task up to his standards, I declined. So, with a zest of excitement, he began the quest to locate the most exclusive doctor in the tristate area. Nothing but the best for him if he had to limit himself to only one set of boobs.

I understood. I was grateful. And scared to death. At the initial consultation, the doctor introduced himself and said, "What can I do for you?"

"She wants breast implants," my husband said.

The doctor didn't respond. Instead, he looked at me. "Stand up for a sec. Come over here." We stood facing each other, and he looked into my eyes. "Tell me what you want," he said.

"I want to look the way I should," I said. "I mean, I guess I want the right size breasts to match the rest of my body." He put his hands on my shoulders and squeezed.

"I'm getting a sense of your frame, your bone structure," he said. Then he ran his hands down my sides and stopped at my hips. Exploring my hip bones for a few seconds, he turned me around with his hands to look briefly at my bum.

"Okay, let's sit," he said. "I only do this procedure by placing the implants under your pectoral muscle. This provides the most natural look, but it's a little more invasive. I'll make a one-inch incision in your armpit. Then, with a tool somewhat like a spatula, I'll splay the muscle away from the bone and insert the empty implant. When the implant is positioned properly, I'll fill it with saline."

Oh my God, splaying muscle from bone? I don't know if I can do this.

"How much does it hurt? How long is the recovery?" I asked.

"The pain varies for everyone. I'm not going to lie; you're going to be sore. You should arrange to stay in bed for three to four days."

Who will look after the kids?

"How big will they be?" my husband asked the doctor.

What if I look like a bimbo? What will people say?

"Will I be able to cook dinner, give my kids a bath, and tuck them in?" I asked.

"They have to be right," my husband said.

"Not for three to four days. Maybe more. Everyone's different," the doctor said.

Walking over to a shelf, the doctor chose three different sizes of breast implants filled with saline from a row of ten and handed them to me. They were jiggly and hard to hold in my hands. I almost dropped them. "Go to a lingerie store together. Take a variety of bra sizes into the change room and try these implants in the bras. See how you look. Come back next week and tell me what you like."

After we left the office, my husband took me directly to a lingerie store. We were in and out in less than ten minutes. He liked the biggest one. I wanted the smallest one.

A week flew by, and we returned to the doctor's office where it turned out the whole exercise of shopping for a boob size was a ruse. The doctor turned to me and said, "Here's the deal. I'm a creator. When you're on my table, in my OR, I'll do what I want. You'll be a walking example of my work." Looking at my husband, he added, "I will put whatever volume of ccs into the implants that I determine is correct. If you don't like it, find someone else." I was speechless and, in a rare moment, so was my husband.

What an egotistical asshole. I'm supposed to surrender my body to surgery with no control over the outcome?! You've got to be kidding!

My husband looked at me.

If I don't do this, he'll have another affair. Or maybe even leave me altogether.

But, if I do, I'll be more attractive, and then, even if he does leave, I'll like myself better.

I turned back to face the doctor. "Okay."

"See my nurse on the way out. She's got a package ready for you. All the instructions are in there. Your surgery date is scheduled for next month. Payment in full is due today."

Oh. Shit just got real. Maybe he won't actually cough up the money. . . .

My husband paid in full without flinching.

I have no idea where the funds came from, but thirty days later, I had big boobs. Luckily, their size is not horrible and they look pretty real. Over time I learned to accept them. But nothing else changed.

I didn't like myself any better; in fact, I liked myself less.

It didn't take much to convince me to get new boobs, did it? I was so desperate to be wanted. Because I was unsure and incapable of even knowing exactly *who* I was, staying true to that woman was incomprehensible to me. There are times when we feel ambivalent, or not really in the mood for doing whatever, that turn out to be enjoyable. That's different. These are situations where we usually would be in genuine agreement. We could say, "I don't really feel like it, but it's important to you, so sure, let's do it!" But, when we agree to do things that we know in our hearts we don't want to do, well, that's how resentment starts.

In our efforts to control whether people like us, we say yes when we want to say no. We agree and go along with others because we want to fit in. We make decisions and do things that we believe will be valued and respected by people we want to impress even when it doesn't feel right. Sometimes we do stupid and irrevocable things to be loved, appreciated, or wanted. We become known as people pleasers. If or when we hear the faint voice telling us that it doesn't feel right, we let the Boss's directives override it.

Sure, other people can be controlling jerks toward us, but we also have the capacity and tendency to be controlling jerks to ourselves. In her sneaky, behind-the-scenes voice, the Boss is yacking away in our heads. Her mission is to keep us afraid. That's how she gets us to do what she wants. All the seemingly little and insignificant times we say yes when we mean no—they all add up. We're so afraid of rejection that we do things, say things—all kinds of things—that we don't really mean, just so people will accept us.

> All the seemingly little and insignificant times we
> say yes when we mean no—they all add up.

We're terrified that if people knew our true nature, if we showed them exactly who we really were and they didn't like us, well, that would be unrecoverable. The Boss teaches us that other people have the power to determine our worth. The factory provides this training. Free of charge.

The Judge in All of Us

Before we get assigned to a management position in the factory, we must undergo judgment training. To pass muster, we'll have to witness, practice, and hone all the skills required of a good judge. The Boss at the Control Factory values judging skills immensely. Whether we learn to judge ourselves or others first is irrelevant because we'll need to get good at both. Either way, learning to assign labels is the first step.

Every label has a positive or negative connotation. There's no middle ground with labels. Even if there's a spectrum to the label, the Boss will make a determination: either good or bad. Fat, thin, stupid, smart, ugly, beautiful, unworthy, deserving. There is a plethora of labels to go around. Further, we get to issue these labels based on whatever criteria we feel like in the moment. The Boss confirms that this is power.

She's also great at showing us how to judge ourselves. By comparing us to everyone else, the Boss encourages us to label ourselves too. And she has an uncanny ability to find and point out evidence to support all the labels she comes up with.

Time for Action

After we assign the labels, it's time to determine what actions are appropriate for our judgment target. This is where the lists (usually in our heads) come into play. Lists are made of all the things other people should and shouldn't do. Once that's done, we assign timelines and dates. Unilaterally, we determine exactly when they should do these things and how long they should take. Next, we specify the necessary outcome, about which there is almost no flexibility. Lastly, we plot our course and strategize tactics to make it happen.

Looking back on the years I raised my boys as a single parent, I now see things differently. When the outcome was positive and the process felt good, it was because I was listening to my heart. My heart told me that my mission as a parent was to raise my kids to be kind, independent, and contribute to society. That's all. That was enough. My heart knew that's what would make them happy. But when I lost my way and subscribed to all the Boss's messages and mandates, that mission was forgotten. It was erased by my fear.

The Boss thinks she knows us better than we know ourselves. And she's even harder on us than she advises us to be on others. She shits on us with her *shoulds* day after day. She doles out unachievable deadlines like a master. And when we miss them or don't perform up to her standards, she helps us assign a new (worse) label. We hate her, but we also believe her.

The Circumstances and Events Departments

The departments of Circumstances and Events have different job descriptions. Our mission here is to create safety, organization, and predictability for ourselves, others, and the world. Because, ya know, our environment and what happens to us are essential to our happiness. It's only possible to feel good if every detail of every little thing is exactly the way we like it, the way it *should* be. We refuse to delegate because nobody is nearly as capable as we are. We work tirelessly to single-handedly determine every schedule and timeline. These positions demand perfection, after all.

The Boss in our head says things like, "That's not a career for girls," "You'll never be happy until you're married," and "Who are you to think you can succeed at that?"

We think we're making ourselves, the world, and everyone else better through our dedication to the factory. Failure is our biggest fear. The Boss will not stand for it. With every unacceptable outcome, she demands new strategies. We are relentless, and oh so very creative, in our mission to orchestrate events or control our environment. We accept the Boss's directives as a surefire way to like ourselves and find happiness. We work hard to learn the ins and outs and the what-have-yous. Resignations are not accepted. It takes more than that to get out of working here, but it is possible.

It's Time to Quit Your Job

The truth is, everything the Boss tells us is a crock of shit. Controlling other people is an illusion and a worthless pursuit. The illusion is that in our efforts to control whatever or whomever, we actually give our power away. We end up giving *them* control over *us*. Here's why.

Controlling other people is an illusion
and a worthless pursuit.

Feeling right feels good. Or so the voice in our head tells us. We erroneously translate right into worthy. The Boss tells us that nobody can be worthy and valuable if they are wrong. But guess what? The Boss at the factory doesn't know everything. In fact, she doesn't know shit from Shinola. The linear thinking of black and white, right and wrong, is rarely helpful and almost always false. Just because we're not right, doesn't make us wrong. In fact, choosing to let go of our *righthood* makes us even more right because right is just a judgment. We can always come up with points to argue our side in an effort to be right. But what's the value in being right? Where does it get us? And, more importantly, what does it cost us?

The Boss tells us not only that we can but also that we must change people. Most of the time, we have good intentions and genuinely want what's best for them. The problem is we think we know what's best. And we don't. Granted, we might have a few good ideas, and it's fair to share those, but only if the person wants to hear them. It's not fair to make the judgment, the decision, or to take actions for an issue that's not ours. Nobody knows what's best for someone else. Only the someone else does. Period.

Regardless of our motivation, the result is the same. Failure to control other people can cause us frustration, anger, worry, guilt, and shame. We end up paying the price, and for what? To make the Boss like us? To show the world how great we are at our jobs? To avoid the feeling of helplessness?

Our ongoing factory work can have a surprising and detrimental impact on us. Eventually, the point will be reached where all attempts at controlling another human will fail, sometimes with disastrous consequences. Then we look around and realize we've just relocated to a different place in Victimtown. We're still here. We've just headed over to the Resentment Parking Lot. Or worse, we've landed our asses in a dark booth at the Guilt & Shame Café.

Retirement

Retirement from the factory is fascinating, and I know I'll always be learning. The Boss is constantly evolving as she tweaks her messages to address our innermost fears around whatever is going on in our lives. We need to keep our shit together, stay strong, and always be learning new ways to stand up to her directives with our heart.

Watching with a new awareness of when and how people perform their duties at the factory is enlightening and often entertaining. Since I've retired, circumstances have emerged more than once when I've been pulled to go back to work for a day or two. The Boss never stops trying to entice us back. Sometimes I get sucked in, but more often my heart voice prevails. It's fun to joke about going back to work when it happens because the work will always be there, and the Boss is ready to remind us how badly it needs to be done. It's not our job to fix other people's problems, especially our children's. For some of us this news will be a relief; for others it may cause more anxiety. It depends on what voice we listen to.

Focusing on ourselves is a choice that provides nourishment and gives space for the yearning seeds to grow. In fact, it took me more than fifty years to stand up to the Boss at the Control Factory. She's hardcore. Even when I wanted to retire, there was an argument, but my heart voice won.

When it comes to controlling others, our heart voice offers these words: "Everything will be okay. They know what's best for them." And when we listen, we can provide loving support while we trust that they will figure it all out.

Change doesn't have to equate with a lack of control. When unexpected things happen to us, it's not because we failed at preventing them. Sometimes, shit happens that we don't deserve. When events don't unfold the way we want, it's not because we did something wrong. Sometimes, shitstorms happen to give us an opportunity to learn or heal. And not everything has an explanation that makes sense in the moment.

Sometimes, shitstorms happen to give
us an opportunity to learn or heal.

Just so ya know, the Ego Arena gets a kickback for recruiting people to work at the factory. Laboring here will either empower us to leave or trap us in Victimtown. Whenever we have problems at work—and problems are inevitable when you work at the Control Factory—we often look for solace somewhere else in town, possibly the Guilt & Shame Café.

CHAPTER 8

The Guilt & Shame Café

*I think the two biggest issues are
world hunger and health, and all the
things that stem from bad food.*
—*Brett Dennen*

One rainy Saturday afternoon, sometime in 1969, my little brother and I were sent to the basement with instructions to play quietly until someone came to get us. I was seven, he was three and a half.

These were our indoor options:

1. Dress up (a hard sell to get my brother's agreement)

2. Hot Wheels (not my favorite)

3. Wooden blocks (kinda fun)

4. Dolls (he would never do it)

5. Hide and seek (needed more kids)

6. TV (cartoons were over for the day)

7. Make a fort (I would have to do all the work)

Number three it was. I dumped several big boxes of blocks onto the floor, and we settled down cross-legged. There were rectangles and squares, cubes and arches, balls, and round columns. Small ones and big ones, in four bright colors. The possibilities for architecture were endless! As we sorted and organized the pieces, we talked about what buildings we'd make, and I described the magnificent town that would be the glorious result of our basement hours. There's a possibility that I was a bit bossy.

Time flew by and the town was developing nicely. Houses sat proudly on two streets; the neighborhood school was built along with an arena. Something about building a store led us to butt heads. Exactly what that something was, I still cannot recall. The result, however, was a three-and-a-half-year-old tantrum that levelled every single building like an earthquake measuring an 8.0 on the Richter scale.

"Look what you did," I said. "What's the matter with you?"

He said nothing.

"You wrecked everything. You have to fix it."

Turning his back to me, he stood his ground silently.

"Listen to me! Do what I say. You have to fix it NOW," I yelled. That got his attention. Turning around, he took a big step forward and swept his foot into the blocks. With all of his might, he sent the biggest pile of town rubble flying—right into my face.

"That's it! I'M TELLING," I said.

The next thing I knew, our mother was there with the wooden spoon, and his pants were coming down. *Oh no! I didn't mean for this to happen.* I heard the smack as the spoon connected with his bare bum. Wincing, I waited for it to be over.

"Get up to your room," our mother said.

Like an aftershock of the earthquake, I watched as my brother defiantly met her eyes directly and stuck his tongue out so far that I was mesmerized by his ability. And then, without breaking eye contact, he moved his head, ever so slightly, from left to right. Not once, but twice. The energy in the room shifted, and I turned away at the last minute to avoid seeing the wooden spoon smack him again.

Why did he do that? Now she's really mad. This wasn't supposed to happen.

I started to cry. He responded with another aftershock. And spoon met bare bum for a third time. *Mommy, STOP! You're hurting him.* Another whack, another aftershock. *This is all my fault. I shouldn't have told on him. I'm a terrible sister.*

Always busy, the Guilt & Shame Café has multiple seating options. The Maître D' evaluates the patrons and decides where each guest will dine. But the Maître D' isn't the only one to have an opinion about our status. The other people hanging out in Victimtown usually have something to say about it too. Some of them are our friends. And on occasion, we let them help decide which section suits us.

Everyone in the café feels bad. Exchanging sympathetic looks, we make small talk and share the nitty-gritty of our wrongdoings, our huge mistakes, and the terrible things that are totally our fault. We commiserate. We're very, very sorry. We're always sorry because everything is our fault. The chair seats are soft and flimsy, and we sink down until our shoulders are level with the tables.

Some of us have real regrets and no matter what we eat, we still feel terrible afterward. Every time we come here, we try something different on the menu, but nothing ever sits well in our stomachs. Yet, we can't help but come back time and again.

Some of us are here because we find comfort in the way the shitty food makes us feel worse. It's the only nourishment we deserve. Most of us don't realize there are other places to eat. Mistakenly, we think this is the only restaurant around. On occasion, we get a table, look at the menu, and decide that we're not ready to eat. We might leave to take a walk on the Denial Trails. Maybe we'll come back later if we get hungry.

On the menu are *bad choice appetizers* and several varieties of *shit sandwiches*. If we become regulars and they know us by name, we develop a complex. The Boss at the factory sends people here to pick up food to go.

At the front, near the windows, there's a large section for those of us who are guilty. The guests on the patio, as well as people walking by, can see us sitting inside. Although we're embarrassed to be here, we know we're not bad people, so it's not the end of the world if someone recognizes us. Tables for two or more are plentiful. And large gatherings are always welcome.

In the very back, beyond a curtain, there's a private room. Only the Maître D' can secure us an invitation to dine here. Far away from the exit door, the lighting is dim, and the only seating option is a private booth. We blush as we enter and are grateful to be incognito. We deserve the seclusion. As we sit alone, with our shoulders slumped and heads hung low, we ruminate excessively.

After the night I dreamt up Victimtown, I viewed some things from my past through a different lens. I didn't like this lens. It was shameful. I could see there were times that I worshipped my victimhood. This new lens revealed that, as a teenager, I took advantage of it. I used it to make myself interesting. I would brag at parties about my Aunt Lynda's murder, how it was still unsolved, and all the trauma (and drama) it had caused. It elevated me when I could speak to the details about the investigation as only an immediate family member could. I had to admit how I actually reveled in the shock value and the fact almost no one could trump my story. It made me feel socially elite. I used it to entertain people and to be liked and to fit in. Society welcomed this. It worked for me. I dishonored my family.

Judging ourselves was learned in the factory and here, in the café, it's our singular obsession. With painstaking detail, we recount every deficiency of our being. The Maître D' judges us too. Never do we talk to anyone else when we're eating. Instead, we replay the stories over and over in our heads, stories that are much too disgraceful to share. We hate to be hiding here, but we know this is where we belong. We just hope nobody will see us.

It makes no difference what we order; there's no point in nourishment anyway. Sometimes, when no one is looking, we scrape our food into a bag and hide it under the table. We are excellent liars.

Self-loathing meatloaf and *dishonored desserts* are served up. The café serves copious amounts of alcohol, both in the front section and the private room. With every meal, the drinks are free, all day, every day! Full bottles are left on the tables so we can serve ourselves. There isn't a drink the bartender doesn't know how to make.

We don't want to eat here in the back room day after day. We can't help it. We long for a satisfying meal, but we have no idea how to find another restaurant. So we keep the tab open, and the years go by. Eventually though, we'll get food poisoning.

The Maître D' hangs out with the factory Boss. They regularly hold masterminds to increase and improve their businesses. When he pops by our table to see how we're doing, the Maître D' says things like, "You're a terrible person," "You should hate yourself, because everyone else does," and even sometimes, "You are worthless."

The age at which we start eating here is different for all of us. The back room isn't just for adults; people of all ages end up in private booths, kids included. There's an old saying: "You are what you eat." When young children start eating here, it becomes a huge challenge for them to learn better eating habits.

I had a friend in my early teens named Sam. She was often sick with stomach issues. Time and again, she had severe and unexplainable stomach pain. They would hospitalize her for a few days, run a bunch of tests that all came back negative, and then release her. And then one day, when we were hanging out in my room, the reason for her stomach pain was revealed. "My stepdad is raping me," she said.

"Oh my God! Have you told your mom?" I asked.

"Yeah. She doesn't believe me, so I'm running away," Sam said. "I told him he'd never touch me again because I'd be gone."

Fed up with my parent's tyranny and wanting to support my friend, I said, "I'm going with you."

We were fourteen. Running away was the only answer. Secretly, we called the Greyhound bus company and asked about fares, destinations, and schedules and decided we'd leave in two days.

We packed light and boarded a Greyhound bus for Buffalo. That was the extent of our plan. It wasn't like we knew anybody in Buffalo. Buffalo was just the farthest we could get with the money we had. And it sounded fun when we chimed, "Buffalo or bust!"

Other than getting far away from home, we had no objective. We didn't talk about what we'd do when we got there or what might transpire along the way and, in no way whatsoever, did we wonder what might happen at the US–Canada border. When we pulled up, a slew of United States Customs & Immigration officers were there to meet us.

An officer boarded our bus and said, "Good day, folks. Birth certificates, please."

He walked down the aisle checking everyone's cards, and when he got to us, we handed ours over with super-sized smiles. He returned them with barely a glance, let alone anything that came close to matching our smiles, and he carried on.

We thought we were in the clear, but when he was finished with the other passengers, he turned around, walked back, and stopped beside us.

"You two. Get your stuff and come with me."

We barely had our feet on the pavement when he motioned for the bus driver to pull out and resume his route.

"You're not old enough," he said.

"What are we supposed to do now?"

"Go home. Back to Canada," he said as he pointed at the bridge.

"How?" we asked.

He started to walk away, then he looked back and said over his shoulder, "Two feet and a heartbeat."

The Peace Bridge is 3,580 feet long. Holding hands, we started making our way as the bridge shook and trembled every time one of the big trucks rolled by. The Canadian customs lady looked amused as we approached her booth on foot.

"Identification please," she said. Again, we handed over our birth certificates. We had them handy. "How long have you been out of the country?" she asked.

"Um, less than an hour," I said.

Customs ladies are no dummies.

"Call your parents," she said. "There's a pay phone in the bar you'll find if you go straight down there for three blocks and then turn right at the gas station for another two. It'll be on your right."

Sam and I looked at each other.

"Off you go. Call them," she said, pointing down the road.

Never leaving my house without a pocketful of quarters from the ever-present safety bowl on my kitchen counter meant that at least we didn't have to ask the bartender for change. I called my dad who didn't even know we were missing. Of course, he left work immediately to drive an hour to pick us up.

My friend returned home and gave up trying to get anyone to believe her. She would reflect on this often throughout her adult years and blame herself for what unfolded afterwards. Her stepdad left her alone from then on. But he didn't stop. He just chose other vulnerable victims. Unable to forgive herself to this day, she berates herself for not trying harder to be believed. As do I. We've both had many meals in the back room of the café. Whatever happened to any of us, whatever we said or did, or whatever we didn't do, if we were eating at the café, we believed everything was our fault.

There have been many detectives assigned to Lynda's case over the years. I was never surprised to see them in my house. Aware of a different energy when I stepped in the door after school, I could feel their presence and would wonder what brought them around this time. My senses were confirmed by the adult huddle at the kitchen table and when I was offered a slice of Nana's fresh pie for a snack *before* dinner.

I'm confident they took their responsibilities seriously and cared deeply about the families of the victims. How could anyone do that job and not feel that way? None of them, however, could provide any of the answers we so desperately craved. I don't think it was from a lack of trying. Or caring. Or working tirelessly. I believe each of them was doing the best they could with the resources they had available at the time, but that didn't make it any easier. My family was living in the Sorrow Swampland.

In times of desperation, people need something—or someone—to hold on to. Families of missing persons tend to hold on to the lead detective. If it's not the lead detective, families assign responsibility to the person providing status updates. Overwhelmed and without considering the impact of their words, family members say things like, "Why can't you do your job?" and "It's your responsibility to find my daughter."

I don't know whether anything like that was uttered by my family members, but it would definitely be understandable. How demoralized the detectives must feel to hear these words. How ashamed they often become when they can't live up to the family's (or their own) expectations. Depending on the circumstances, they can begin to doubt their professional abilities and even their own fundamental worth.

One detective in particular, Dennis Alsop, had a long and distinguished career. Although he was successful in solving many heinous crimes, three murder cases eluded him: Jackie English, Soraya O'Connell, and Lynda White. He never stopped working on these cases, even in retirement. After he passed away in 2012, his son found a cardboard box containing all of his investigative notes along with his personal theories about these unsolved cases that occurred in the late 1960s. His extensive records and thoughtful interpretations were a tribute to all the detectives of his time who relied solely on their minds and their wits to solve murders without the technology employed today. They had to find answers before surveillance cameras, DNA testing, or information databases existed. In an interview, Alsop's son Dennis Jr. said, "He left this stuff and he left it intentionally. He never forgot it was here."[1] Victimtown isn't only where victims of crimes end up. Detectives spend time there too.

Al Fresco Dining

The Guilt & Shame Café also has a patio. These outside seats, however, are reserved for quick eaters. With a limited menu, the food arrives in short order, and there's an expectation that you'll enjoy your meal without lingering. If you want to hang out, you'll need to move inside.

Sitting here, we wallow for a bit and feel genuinely sorry for our role in whatever happened. We're not quite ready to face facts or to confront the people that know what we did. We're working up to it, though. While we're eating, we do our best to not hear what the Maître D' is saying inside.

The folks on the patio have all made a pretty big mistake. Some are doozies with life-altering consequences, while others are less significant. United in our collective feeling of misgiving, we exchange sympathetic looks. But here, outside in the fresh air, after we share our stories and express our sorrow, we brainstorm and strategize about making amends. Doing our best to eat quickly, we know we've come to the right place.

The most important element of eating here is to digest our meal properly. This is how we learn from our mistakes and become a better person. We all can benefit from a meal here from time to time. Feeling revitalized, and with a plan for sorting out our shit, we go on our way.

The Maître D's voice isn't nearly as loud from our seats on the patio. Our heart voice speaks with words of comfort like, "You did the best you could," "You're not a bad person," and "Do what you can to make it up to them."

As I passed through my teenage years and matured, I became more of a private victim, and the telling of Lynda's tragedy diminished. But the mentality prevailed. The Maître D' confirmed that I was a terrible person, while the Boss continued to tell me that I was responsible for my parents' happiness and I was doing a shitty job. All of which substantiated the fact that I was, therefore, unlovable. All of my fears were justified. Every. Single. One.

Eating at the Guilt & Shame Café will either make us healthier or make us very, very sick, depending on where we sit and what we eat. With no wait lists for any of the sections, there's always tables available. The Maître D' wants to fill up the back room. Where we ultimately end up sitting is directly proportionate to how loud our heart voice responds. Regardless of which section that is, it's always where we already know we belong.

CHAPTER 9

The Resentment Parking Lot

The heart is like a garden.
It can grow compassion or fear,
resentment or love.
What seeds will you plant there?
—*Jack Kornfield*, Buddha's Little Instruction Book

N ot long after my nana's mental breakdown, Bampa had a massive stroke. It didn't matter that he was only in his fifties and very healthy up to that point; the damage to his brain was severe. But then, something miraculous happened. Nana instantly became well. To me, it seemed like magic. What really took place was that the urgent need for her support in this new crisis gave her purpose again. It was essential for her to be healthy to advocate for her husband's care.

Bampa spent a year in the hospital and was fortunate to benefit from a further year in an excellent rehab facility nearby. The stroke left him paralyzed on the entire right side of his body. Determined, he made amazing progress relearning how to walk, eat, and everything else that able-bodied people take for granted. The stroke also resulted in a condition called aphasia, which occurs when the bleeding in the brain damages the parts that control language and communication. It can affect the ability to speak, write, type, and read. So, basically, it can inhibit or eliminate the ability to communicate with words. Imagine the nightmare of living a never-ending, 24/7 life of charades. In the beginning, he couldn't say anything, but eventually he could get out a word or two. Never again would he tell us any of the long and hilariously detailed stories for which he was known.

The day came for Nana and my parents to plan for his return home. It was decided that our two families should live together. As the first grandchild, I held a special place in his heart, and I adored him. I was proud to be responsible for his title of Bampa. The stroke couldn't take away his keen sense of humor as he found new ways of nonverbal expression. He developed a variety of very meaningful looks. His wink became famous. Verbally, however, he had only one word down pat. It was a common word. One word, a vehicle through which he could communicate his feelings easily and with precision. A word with the largest variety of connotations, depending on the emphasis, facial expression, and other body language. The word was SHIT. It was the only word he could get out any old time he wanted. And he used it a lot. All day, every day, he said "shit" to mean everything under the sun. And he didn't get in trouble for it. This was, without a doubt, the most hilarious development. I like to think that he chose that word because it made me laugh so hard. It was better than cartoons. It certainly lightened the vibe for everyone else too, especially those coming to our house for the first time.

I was really excited to live with Nana and Bampa. Finding the right house was very challenging because we needed a main floor bedroom with a full bathroom to accommodate my grandparents, as well as three bedrooms for our family. In the end, we renovated my grandparents' house, the home my mom grew up in. A bedroom and bathroom were built as an addition to the main floor, and at the end of September, three weeks into my fourth-grade school year, we moved in.

Nana moved downstairs to the new room. My parents took over my grandparents' bedroom. My brother got the original boys' room. And I was given Lynda's room. It was big and bright and had not one but two closets! It was much nicer than my old room, and I was eager to settle in.

My dad brought up five or six boxes and set them on the floor for me. I opened the first one to find my books. I looked around. There was a bookcase on one wall, but it was already full. I didn't see anywhere else to put them, so I shoved it aside and opened the next box: clothes. I opened the first closet. It was full. I opened the second closet, and there was a bit of space but not enough. I turned around and studied the room. It was as if Tabatha had wiggled her nose and transformed everything, like in my favorite TV show *Bewitched*. That's when I noticed Lynda's favorite stuffed animals were staring back at me from the bed. I remember thinking, *Our pajama party friends look lonely and sad.*

Her sports medals and ribbons hung proudly on the bulletin board. A jewelry box sat on the dresser with a few of her bracelets hanging out. A half-read book was covered in dust on the bedside table.

Then it hit me like a brick wall.

This is Lynda's room.

It looked like she had gone off to university and would be home soon for a weekend visit. But would she?

I sat on her bed, taking it all in.

What am I supposed to do with her things?

I wanted her to come home. Desperately. We all did. But it had been three years now. Was that even possible?

This isn't your bedroom. You shouldn't be here.

I used to have sleepovers in this room, but she was with me. Now it was just me, and I wasn't sure what to do. I felt like an intruder.

Should I move her things? Do I pack them up? I can't ask my parents; it'll make my mom wail again. And what if Nana comes up and sees that the room has changed?

I started to cry.

I wished I could wiggle my nose like Tabitha and make it all disappear.

Pulling my thumb out of my mouth, I shoved all of my boxes into the corner and walked out of the room, closing the door behind me.

I wish we didn't move here. But what I want doesn't matter anyway. Nobody cares about me.

How Resentment Starts

Not being able to ask for what we need or want cultivates resentment. If this sounds familiar to you, you may have spent some time in the Resentment Parking Lot. This underground parking lot has multiple entrances from the street level. Old crumbling cement ramps lead us down. Level after level, this parking lot is crammed full. Expensive cars, old jalopies, motorcycles, trucks, vehicles pulling trailers, and even bicycles park here.

It's often hard to get a spot, but we're relentless. Down and around we go, searching in the dim light until we find a place to park. We pull in, take a deep breath, and start thinking about what happened. We think and we think, and we think. The event could have been last week, last year, or twenty years ago. It doesn't matter; we're able to readily bring back the details with an uncanny (and occasionally embellished) clarity. Details of past relationships, deep hurts, betrayals, unkind words, and every single rejection. None of which was our fault.

While everyone is welcome, the fees are not posted, so we enter without any idea of how expensive it is to park here. Having said that, it is fun to hang out and shoot the shit. We're having such a good time that the cost never enters our mind. Sitting in our cars, we roll down our window and commiserate with the guy in the car next to us. We're all eager to share our grudges. Groups of people get out of their cars and are naturally drawn to each other to take turns at grudge-telling events. Long lists of resentments circulate.

With a serious demeanor, the lot Attendant makes his rounds and adamantly says things like, "What they did is completely unforgivable" and "You're better than them."

Understanding and comradery are thick in this parking lot. Everyone can relate to how the other feels. Take my mom, for example. All my friends confirmed my right to resent her enforcing all those weird rules growing up. It's a close-knit club, this parking lot, and the sound of our ranting echoes up into the streets. Not infrequently, there's a competition about who had the shittiest things happen to them. More than a few times, I won. But winning here has its price. The air in the lot is filled with toxic, bitter fumes. Headaches, muscle tension, and nausea prevail. Unaware, or just not caring, we continue to talk to whomever will listen through our clenched jaws.

We're genuinely proud to be seen here, even though our emotions can sometimes get out of control. In our frustration, we can be short-tempered and occasionally hostile. But our behavior is justified; it's both understandable and acceptable. Standing on the hood of our car, we shout to be heard above the rest. The world must know we've been tragically wronged! Every time we share, we feel our emotions revving up. "That asshole," we say, "I can't *believe* they did that to me." We don't understand, let alone admit, the part of us that's actually jealous of their ability to stand up for themselves. And if we get really revved up, our bitterness sends us running out to fuel up at the Anger Gas Station. And where we go from there is anybody's guess.

While we're parked here, we believe we have a kind of power over the person we hold the grudge against. It's a good feeling and we like it. A lot. We laugh heartily at the people who did us wrong, and we pity them for their inadequacies. We would *never* do what they did. It's irrelevant if this person has apologized. Any attempts to make amends for their wrongdoing fall short of the mark in our mind. "Really? You think that makes up for it?"

People here sometimes wish for events ten times as bad to befall the perpetrator because, well, they totally deserve it. Karma is often discussed, and we can't wait for the day when they get theirs. That's when we will have won. Won't it be great? That'll be a day to celebrate. WE ARE SO RIGHT!

We get a thrill out of parking here. It feeds our warped sense of self-worth as it makes us feel superior. We feel righteous. We don't taste the bitterness at all. Not even a little bit. After a bad day working at the factory, we might stop here on the way home to vent. Our complaints are approved and justified by our pals. Nobody here wants anyone else to leave, so we keep the commiserating going. If we're not seen here for a while, our comrades will start to wonder what's going on with us.

Over time, and with repetitive telling of the same event, our stories tend to morph. Rarely do we minimize our experience. Almost always, it becomes worse. Much worse. More disastrous, more heinous. More condemning.

And if we think about leaving, the Attendant will say, "You're letting them win. Is that what you really want?" or "Fine. Go ahead. Just try to move on." The Attendant will snicker when you walk away, and he'll keep calling out to you.

The Revenge Parking Lot: For Long-Term Stays

If we show up here with a full tank of gas from the Anger Gas Station, the Attendant might direct us to the long-term parking section. That's the Revenge Parking Lot. A lot of us think about it, but not everyone has actually been there. We've heard that it's climate-controlled with wide parking spaces and electrical hookups. It sounds enticing, and we believe that a vindicated sticker will be issued when we exit. Although we might fantasize about parking there, and we might even make a plan, we also have an inkling about how dangerous it can be. It's not until we leave and get the bill that we'll have to come to terms with just how much it cost us.

Some of the statements get lost in the mail and we don't receive them for years. The interest that can accrue has the power to bankrupt us.

The High-Rise Parking Lot: For Short-Term Parking

Okay, I get it. Some of you may be wondering what's wrong with holding grudges. There is a general consensus in the lot that grudges are fine as long as we don't go into the Revenge Lot. Parking our cars in short-term parking and taking some time out to stretch our legs isn't necessarily a bad thing. Or if we need a quick reset, we can choose a high-rise parking lot that offers more space to air our grievances.

The truth is, being parked for any great length of time doesn't serve our self-worth in any way. The Attendant also upholds the three shitty beliefs. We know from our previous factory jobs that what other people do is not our concern. We're only in charge of ourselves. The mean-spirited acts that people indulge in are not about us. People who act out in those ways are hurting terribly inside. They are in great pain. Their own pain. There's no excuse for cruelty. However, the cost of holding grudges and resentments must be acknowledged. We can all afford different cars and different lifestyles. It's a personal choice as to how and where we decide to park our vehicles.

A short stopover in the high-rise lot allows us to air our beefs and be done with it. Taking the time to sit with our feelings enables us to get them out of our system. Forgiveness is considered here. When we can walk away in peace from whatever experience, whatever person caused us harm, we strengthen our heart voice and it will affirm that, "It's okay to let it go, to be happy, and move on."

Parking in the Resentment Lot will either make us kinder and more compassionate or more bitter and judgmental—unless, of course, we're not ready to address the issue at all.

CHAPTER 10

The Denial Trails

People spend entire lifetimes trying to avoid
the things that have already happened.

—Silvia Hartmann

About six months after we moved into my grandparents' house, my mom told me to get in the car. Nana was driving with my mom in the passenger seat. Seatbelt laws were not yet in effect. I jumped in and flung my elbows over the back of the front seat. With my face only inches from theirs, I asked, "Where are we going?"

"To pick something up," Mom said.

"What?" I asked.

"Just something."

"What something?"

"Just *something.*"

This last answer was delivered with *the tone*. I knew this tone. It's a popular parent tone. I'd tried it out a few times on my younger brother. It's the tone that meant STOP ASKING ME QUESTIONS.

Frustrated, I sat down on my seat. I stared at the back of my mother's head and played a game of odds in my mind wondering if I'd get an answer. Nothing. I tried to catch her attention in the rearview mirror by making saucer eyes and prune lips and rapid head wiggles. Still nothing. In defeat, and with a dramatic pout, I sent my mother a childish "F you" by doing an about-face. Up on my knees, with my chin on two hands, I stared out the back windshield. In my petulance, I stayed that way for the entire drive. When the car finally stopped, and when I turned around, I saw that we were parked in someone's driveway. I'd never been there before, and I was pretty sure that Nana and Mom hadn't either. They looked at each other without words, but there was a meaning in the air. It felt like a secret. I could hardly contain my curiosity, but I was too afraid to say anything.

My mother got out of the car and went to the door. Almost immediately, she returned with a small paper bag. It was the same kind of paper bag that my school lunch was packed in, just not as full.

What's in it? I wanna know.

My fear of antagonizing her and getting punished, however, kept me quiet. Nana's hands were on the wheel, but the car stayed put even after Mom got back in.

Staring straight ahead, without looking at anyone, Nana said, "Don't touch it."

"Right," Mom said.

They sat in silence, and their glances bounced from the brown paper lunch bag to each other and then out the windshield, from the brown paper lunch bag, to each other, and then out the windshield. On round two of this glancing game, I caught on to their discomfort. That's when my mother picked up the brown paper bag, reached back, and put it onto the seat beside me.

"Don't touch it," she said to me.

What?? What do you mean? Why can't I touch it?

There was no way I could ask anything. I didn't even want to know anymore because now I was terrified of that bag. And it was on the seat right beside me! What I really wanted to do was play the hot potato game. I wanted to throw that sucker right back at her, but I was way too scared to touch it.

What if we go around the corner and it falls off the seat? Oh my God . . . what if we go around a corner and it slides over and touches me?

I decided to pretend it wasn't there. I fixed my gaze out the side window, and very soon the brown paper bag no longer existed. As my anxiety lessened, my breathing returned to normal.

Then, without a word, Nana put the car in reverse and backed out.

I thought we were going home. And it looked that way for a few turns, but then we headed in a different direction. About a block away I realized we were going to a place already familiar to me.

Oh NO! I wish I didn't come. I hate them. This nightmare will never end.

We'd arrived at the police station.

From toddlers to seniors, people from every walk of life have hiked on the Denial Trails at some time or another. If we hear someone we know is in Victimtown and we can't find them, there's a good chance they're on these trails. Somewhere.

With route maps translated into multiple languages, this trail system offers an extensive variety of hikes and activities. Hundreds of workers cover every trail from end to end with responsibilities much like that of a concierge. Except here, they're called Dirtbags.

Preferring to overstaff, the Trails Association's number-one priority is to provide whatever experience hikers are looking for. Without exception, every hiker's needs are accommodated. The cost of labor is inconsequential. The slippery slopes are not mentioned—and there are many. Excitedly, the Dirtbags welcome one and all with these reassuring words: "You don't have to think about that issue anymore. Whatever it takes to ease your pain is good for you."

We all show up here to avoid something. It could be a difficult task, our worries, conflict, certain people, shit that's happening, our dreams, the consequences of our actions, tragic events, what we believe, being vulnerable, facing facts, expectations, doing something we might regret, how we look, being excluded, tough conversations, what we really want, current problems, judgment, bad memories, who we really are, what people think of us, our fears, what's not happening, having to provide answers, facing our shame, being wrong, admitting something we've done, the truth, our inability to control something, our faults, needing something or someone, owning our stories, things we can't change, our bad habits, disappointment, reality, or even the voices in our head. Phew. Long sentence.

It boils down to this: We usually end up on the Denial Trails to avoid difficult feelings like pain, grief, shame, rejection, failure, hate, embarrassment, hopelessness, guilt, or anger. It's hard to feel that shit. Nobody likes it. You may be surprised to learn that we also come here to avoid great feelings like acceptance, joy, success, accomplishment—even love.

With such a vast number of reasons to hike, it's easy to see why people of all ages, from every walk of life, have spent time on the Denial Trails. For some, when shit happens, this is their first stop in Victimtown. Others walk over from the Guilt & Shame Café if they don't like the food, or from the Control Factory when work's not going well, or the Anger Gas Station if they run out of fuel while driving around. The folks that have been living in Victimtown for a while, well, most of them schedule regular hikes in their planners. The Dirtbags know them by name and provide a custom experience. Evening strolls are very popular with this group.

At the trailhead stands a ginormous building with ornate wooden doors that open to massive rooms containing walls and walls of shelves. The Issue Building. This is where we drop off our issue, so we can hike without having to carry it around. It's the hassle-free way to fully enjoy the trails and everything they offer.

The Dirtbag on door duty decides how each issue will be stored. Boxes of all sizes are available. Heavily padded, some issue boxes are built to protect the most crippling problems. Back-up boxes are lead-lined to prevent messy issues from leaking out. Not all issues are stored in closed boxes, however; some deserve a pedestal.

There's often a disconnect between the size and type of box the gatekeeper chooses versus what the hiker believes is the right fit. For example, a hiker might think their issue is kind of insignificant, that it'll fit in a small box. The gatekeeper, however, might think that the issue demands a much bigger box and a lot of padding. The opposite is also true. Some people are taken by surprise to see their issue placed in a huge box. "Oh. Wow. I didn't think it was that big of a deal," they say. The Dirtbag at the gate determines which issues are placed on a pedestal, which sometimes leaves hikers in disbelief. Here's the bottom line: Issues are complicated. The Dirtbags boast about their great proficiency and accuracy at judging issues. The handbook for working here was written by the Boss. A sign posted by the Trails Association reads, "All Dirtbag decisions are final."

Patient with most hikers, Dirtbags hear the same question over and over: "Hey . . . um . . . any chance that, instead of storing it, you can just dispose of this issue for me?"

"Feel free to leave it here as long as you'd like," the Dirtbags say. Most hikers don't notice the small sign on the building that says, "TEMPORARY STORAGE ONLY. ALL ISSUES MUST BE RETRIEVED UPON EXIT. NO EXCEPTIONS." And if they do, the Dirtbag adds, "Don't worry about it! You're in the right place!"

Then he hands us an empty backpack.

"Here you go. There's lots to see and do on the trails. Have a great time."

So, we slap the backpack on and head out. What we don't see are all the ambulances lined up like taxis behind the Issue Building. The transfer of injured hikers to the Epiphany Hospital is nonstop. Search and rescue crews are also kept busy with urgent calls from friends and families in Freedomville. But we don't notice any of that when we hand over our issues and hop on a trail.

In 2018, I flew to Hawaii for vacation. My boyfriend and I rented a condo on the big island. On a quiet Saturday morning, about a week into our trip, I was in the kitchen packing our lunch for a day of adventure while he was watching basketball on TV. Out of nowhere, an incredibly loud alarm started going off. It was a sound I'd never heard before. For the life of me, I could not figure out where it was coming from. It was the strangest thing. This obnoxious sound had to stop! Frantically, I searched for the source. When I finally located it, I was shocked to find that it was coming from my phone. *What the hell?* I'd never seen a phone screen this bright. I read slowly: "BALLISTIC MISSILE THREAT INBOUND TO HAWAII. SEEK IMMEDIATE SHELTER. THIS IS NOT A DRILL."

Huh. Wow. This is weird.

My brain started processing. *How on earth did my kids find this joke app that could do this to my phone?*

With boys aged twenty-six and twenty-eight, this was just the kind of humor I was used to. *Let's get Mom while she's on vacation. Ha ha ha.*

Laughing at the joke and marveling at their ingenuity, I walked in to show Bob my phone. I stopped in my tracks when I saw the TV. The red ticker that they reserve for breaking news was running across the screen. The exact. Same. Message. Bob looked confused. I showed him my phone. We stared at each other, speechless.

Holy shit. This is not a joke.

The reality of our situation began to sink in along with the realization that there was nowhere to seek shelter. We were on a volcanic island. Where would we go? There were no basements, no shelters, and obviously, no time to leave the island. It was your basic conundrum of possibly deadly proportions.

SHIT!

"Let's go to the beach," I said. "Right away. If there's a missile coming, I wanna disintegrate instantly. I really, really don't want to die the slow burn."

My boyfriend agreed.

"Maybe we should text our kids," I said.

I quickly sent a group text to my boys: "Hey. Got a weird message about an incoming missile. Not sure what's going on but just want to say that I love you."

Almost immediately, my oldest, and very pragmatic, son wrote back: "Well, Momma Dukes, if you're going to get F*&king nuked, at least you're in Hawaii."

Hm. That's a little harsh . . . I mean, yeah, he's been here and knows this beauty firsthand, and he knows that it's my favorite place on earth, but REALLY?

I sat with it for a minute, and then I saw it.

Ah. Yes. He's absolutely right.

There are a million worse ways to go. And then my younger, worldly son chimed in: "Hey, Momma Bear, don't worry. North Korea can't hit anything they're aiming at."

Well. Alrighty then. Ah . . . what amazing offspring I have!

But time was ticking. And there was none to waste.

Oh God, I can't believe this is happening.

We raced down three flights of stairs and jumped into the jeep. Driving in silence, I was mentally on the Denial Trails and found tremendous reassurance from the Dirtbag's voice in my head.

Smoke a joint. Have a drink. Stare at the ocean and don't think about it.

In addition to the Dirtbag narrating your visit, the Denial Trails are well-marked with wide, groomed paths. Their popularity alone proves that these trails offer world-class routes. The map posted at the trailhead offers two choices: We can select the two-mile route or the extended five-mile route. At certain points, hikers need to make a choice about which path to take. They can switch routes or continue looping around. There are also many opportunities for hikers to veer off and explore unique views and enjoy different activities along the trail, but danger looms around almost every corner. You might think you know where you're going, but conditions can change very quickly. Mudslides occur when you're least expecting it. Directional signs are wrong. And nothing here is as it seems. Those are just the tip of the iceberg when it comes to the dangers on the trails. There are no time limits imposed, which is irrelevant as we usually lose track of time anyway. Whether we hike on the Denial Trails for a short walk or a lifetime, the only safe way out is the way we came in.

Dirtbags are stationed frequently along the trails. Easily recognized by their flannel shirts and unkempt appearance, they possess a wealth of knowledge about hiking, activities, and the terrain. They give advice constantly and with authority.

The trails are unique in that truth doesn't exist there. Reality is skewed, and everyone lies. About everything. And nobody cares. The Dirtbags will reassure us every step of the way that we are fine, all is good, and there's nothing to worry about. They excel at enabling us to avoid thinking about whatever issue we dropped off. In fact, they strive to ensure that we don't feel anything we don't want to.

On the two-mile route, the trail is fresh and uncomplicated. With some decent views, it offers enough activity choices for most people. Hikers who saw the sign and accepted the storage policy for their issue generally find the time spent on this shorter route to be restorative and helpful. They only need a water bottle and light snack. Without sleeping or cooking gear, their packs are ultralight, and they can generally navigate their own way out.

There's always the chance that when they reach the choice point, however, that they might decide to loop around again or get lured into seeing what the five-mile route offers. The Dirtbags are constantly encouraging us to stay with suggestions.

"Life is fun and easy here."

"The longer routes have the best views! Besides, all the other hikers want you to stay."

The five-mile route is deceiving. It starts out pleasantly enough, but slowly, the terrain changes. Without realizing it, we soon find ourselves having to tread a bit more carefully as we trudge along, still excited for our next distraction. The trails offer endless activity choices. Willing to provide whatever we want to keep us busy, the Dirtbags provide enticements with one purpose: to get hikers addicted. Our wish is their command. Things like exercise stations with barbells and personal trainers, lounge areas with the most comfortable recliners to settle in and watch every Netflix series available, every new-release movie, and every TV channel in the entire world are there for the taking. Workstations where we can pick up a laptop are everywhere. We can throw laptops in our backpacks and look for a spot to relax and check out the links to shopping sites we never knew existed. Free alcohol is available whenever we desire, but we must take the bottle with us. Drinking on the trails is expected. It's here on the trails that we often do things that we've never done before. Substances of every type imaginable are readily supplied. And we're beyond grateful to have zero time for reflection.

Dirtbags love it when the trails are packed. As master negotiators, they encourage cowboy camping, which entails sleeping under the stars. Happily, they give us sleeping bags and cooking sets and even straps to tie it all on to our packs. They're the best hosts ever, and they entertain us with stories of how easy life is on the trails in their attempts to seduce us into becoming through-hikers. They offer us the gift of a "trail name," a special moniker to use while we're there to help us dissociate from our issues. Addiction abounds with the campers on the Denial Trails.

Halfway along the five-mile route we're met with the final hill, a stressful push to the top. The peak is within reach. Anticipating feelings of happiness and joy, we feel the weight of our packs more than ever as we take the last few steps. Then, much to our dismay, we realize it was a false peak. We take in the vista anyway. For a brief instant, we think about how long we've been hiking this trail and begin to wonder what we should do next.

We might have a niggling feeling that going down the trail will be harder than going up. There was no time to think about that when we were busy having so much fun, but we're starting to miss some people in our lives and wonder what's going on in the rest of the world. None of us relish the thought of having to pick up our issue on the way out. That's assuming we saw the sign or that somebody told us about it. If not, we're in for a bit of a shock. Nevertheless, the Dirtbags don't want to see us go. They'll offer a timely comment like, "Are you sure you know the way back?" Looking down, we see how punishing it will be to give way to all the people trudging uphill. Bushwhacking on the back side is our only other option.

As we ponder our next steps, the Dirtbags continue to spew advice.

> "Have some drinks and you'll feel better."
> "Your issue is impossible to figure out."
> "Just keep busy so you don't have to think about it."
> "If you really want, I can give you directions to the Swamp."

I spent most of my life hiking a variety of routes on the trails as I bounced around in Victimtown from one place to another. The Dirtbags knew me so well they could anticipate my needs: Oyster

Bay Sauvignon blanc, Netflix and a couch, seventy-hour workweeks, a new house to renovate, Veuve, and less and less contact with my friends and family. Maybe a new Peloton bike or an online fashion shopping spree.

They even began to tailor their messages with precision: "Nobody cares about you. You've got way too many issues in storage. Besides, it's too late to get them out now. You'll never be able to handle it."

One thing was true: I did have a lot of issues in storage. The one that grew the biggest over the years was Lynda's disappearance and all the subsequent events that occurred in my childhood. With those issues (and more) stored tightly in boxes, I was easily convinced by the Dirtbags that endless hiking and cowboy camping was the best I could do.

That is, until one day when my Netflix access was interrupted, and I made my way down and jumped into one of the ambulances. I remember a Dirtbag yelling at me, "What are you doing? I'll get you whatever you want, and you can figure out your shit here on the trail!"

To which I said, "YOU DON'T KNOOWWW ME."

And I said it exactly like Brené Brown.

Determined hikers eventually make it back to the trailhead on their own. Inevitably, the Dirtbag on duty will retrieve their issue. Some issues become moldy and dirtier the longer they're left boxed up. Others take on a life of their own in storage; they grow and morph, and we're shocked when we see them again. And then there are some that are in pretty much the same state as they were when we dropped them off, which is usually the best-case scenario. Only once in a blue moon do the issues improve with age.

In case you're thinking of pulling a fast one on the trails, I should let you know that all attempts to convince a Dirtbag that your issue really belongs to someone else will fail. Exhausted and desperate hikers often try to offload their shit by offering huge incentives to anyone willing to take their issue. And if you come across a hiker taking a break from their high-level job at the Control Factory, well, they might agree to do just that. Be forewarned: If you hand over your issue, you'd better be ready to deal with the outcome.

On occasion, the odd hiker tries to sneak out without taking their issue, but the Dirtbags are fast and tenacious. Even if it takes years, or an entire team of Dirtbags, without fail the issue is always returned to its proper owner.

The hikers that make it off the trail on their own resign themselves to taking responsibility for all of their issues. They often do this in the face of hearing a very sarcastic "Good luck with that" from a Dirtbag.

Lots of hikers want to drop off their heavy backpack before they leave. They don't want the reminder of their time on the trails, and the Dirtbags are happy to take it, but only if we stay too. The stuff we accumulate while we're hiking, that stuff is ours now, just like our original issues. We can choose to deal with that stuff ourselves, too. We can accept it all. We must. Because it's ours.

The Denial Trails will always be full of Dirtbags pushing and pulling us toward more treacherous routes and farther distances. Bushwhacking is the most dangerous endeavor. That's where the passages are thoroughly phony, your mind plays tricks, and reality is completely skewed. Chasing false peak after false peak, all sense of direction is eventually lost. In the end, whenever the end happens for the hiker, at the last minute, they will know.

Stepping Off the Trails

Once in a while, for no apparent reason and completely out of left field, life throws us into a shitstorm of issues. In hindsight, we might see clues about how this happened, but sometimes a shitstorm hits us like a rogue wave, without warning. No matter how it happens, I want you to know that there are always other options besides going for a long hike on the trails. Listening to our heart voice helps us be less afraid. When you can be gentle with yourself, breathe, take things a step at a time, and seek out the support you need to help you process your issues in a healthy way, you'll be less likely to end up on the trails.

Healthy Hikes

There are times when we just need to set aside an issue while we gather our wits. While we remain realistic about it, sometimes a short stroll on the trails isn't always the worse thing. When we're doing the best we can, when we're fully prepared to pick up our issue in a day or two, I want you to know that it's okay to take a short time to adjust to whatever shit has happened. But you'll need to be cautious because none of us can stop the Dirtbags from talking altogether, so it's critical that we not put any stock in what they have to say.

A short break from our issue might help us summon the strength and find the support we need to tackle our problem. A short walk may lead us to discover that we're exactly where we need to be. The trails, and all the places in Victimtown, offer us opportunities for growth. Victimtown offers gifts, even on the trails. The gifts are found in the awareness of where you are and in the honesty with yourself about why you're there. And when you listen to your heart, you'll be less inclined to succumb to the Dirtbags' tactics to keep you there.

Obviously, I didn't die from a ballistic missile. Thirty-eight minutes after the initial warning, another text announced that the threat was false. False. As in, someone just made a mistake. No biggie. Of course, it was good news. We got to live. We carried on with our vacation and put the whole thing behind us.

Many years later, during a therapy session, this story came out. My therapist was astounded. She couldn't believe I hadn't told her about this—that I'd left this issue in storage for so long. She told me that the fact that I'd believed my death to be imminent, even for only thirty-eight minutes, was not a small issue. Apparently, this event had a significant impact on my mental health. Who knew? Turns out, I'd only exasperated matters by not taking the time to feel the feelings I had at the time. It was much easier to ignore my fear, forget about it entirely, and to just soldier on. With my new lens, I think the scare taught me that you never know how long you've got. Now I can see how that event fertilized the seeds of my yearnings. And it allowed me to understand that issues in storage continue to affect us while we're busy doing whatever we're doing on, or off, the trails.

My issues filled a pretty big suitcase, which I had no choice but to bring with me when I flew to The Place. A few of them hadn't changed; most of them I couldn't yet look at, but the ones that I briefly examined had grown and were decidedly yucky.

The Denial Trails may be a beaten path, but it isn't the only passage to hike. Many wonderful trails are out there along with inspiring reasons to hike them. Our heart voice knows which ones are best for us. I still have a few issues. I expect I always will. The difference is that now I've got the strength to carry them, and by giving them lots of love, they get lighter every day.

Time on the Denial Trails can be therapeutic or catastrophic. While the distinction and the defining line for what is therapeutic can be a little different for each of us, catastrophic is pretty clear. Catastrophic can keep us on the trails, land us in the Epiphany Hospital, or lead us to other places in Victimtown, like the Anger Gas Station.

CHAPTER 11

The Anger Gas Station

Wherever you go, you take yourself with you.

—Neil Gaiman, The Graveyard Book

Eventually, I did learn the details behind the paper lunch bag pickup in my Aunt Lynda's abduction case. Construction of a building had been underway a few miles from our house, and while scooping up a bucketful of dirt, a bulldozer driver noticed something odd mixed in with the soil. It piqued his curiosity—so much so that he shut off his machine, lowered the bucket, got out, and walked around to pick this thing out and examine it. Why he did this, we'll never know. It was an old wallet. The only thing inside was an identification card with the owner's name, Lynda White. He recognized the name, because her case made headlines in the newspapers off and on for many years. I don't know why he didn't call the police; he must've known our family, because he put it in a brown paper lunch bag and called our house.

This new evidence started another big round of attention that led to speculations and headlines once again. This time, though, my parents had a new strategy for the angst it would cause my grandparents. Their solution was me.

My new job was to sit on the front porch every day after school and wait for the newspapers to be delivered. With a pair of scissors and instructions to cut out all the articles relating to Lynda, her case, or the wallet, I sat by myself (pissed off, obligated, and responsible) on our concrete porch and ate my after-school snack.

It doesn't matter what you want. Just suck it up and get the job done.

I would do anything to make them less sad. My careful cuts produced oddly shaped holes in the newspaper pages. I wondered what my grandparents would think when they saw the holes. Surely, they would know what was in each one. As per my instructions, I would gently place the cut-out articles in the box provided to me for this purpose. The Lynda Box. There were already so many clippings in there.

They're the grown-ups. Why can't they do this?

It wasn't until a full week went by without a mention in any of the newspapers that I was relieved of my post. After the police finished their analysis of the wallet, it was determined to be only an old trinket from Lynda's childhood, something that she'd likely lost while playing in that field many years ago. It had no relevance whatsoever to her disappearance. What are the odds?

Before Lynda disappeared, I was a confident child. I talked to strangers at every opportunity, always eager to share my observations and ideas. I asked for everything I needed and wanted and sometimes threw tantrums if I didn't get it. The only thing that bugged me about myself was my big ears because kids made fun of them. Mostly it was okay, though, because my long hair hid them, except when they poked out. I wasn't self-conscious about anything else. I was happy and silly, and I felt safe and loved.

Then I watched all the adults in my world become more helpless with every day that passed without answers or Lynda's return. I knew I was on my own. I armored up to face the world by myself, keeping my anger inside to avoid upsetting my already seriously upset family.

To this day, I almost never watch the news or read a newspaper. I didn't know it then, but forty years later, I would once again become the keeper of the Lynda Boxes (now plural). They contain so much more than newspaper clippings. Just the sight of them, let alone holding them or exploring the contents, evokes an intense emotional response in me that's run the gamut of every single place in Victimtown. Over the years, I've handled them many times, including, but not limited to, moving them multiple times with my mom to another house, lugging them up from the basement so new detectives could familiarize themselves with the contents, opening them to deposit additional documents, dumping them at my uncle's house and running away after my mom's stroke, and finally, coming to terms with the gift of Lynda's role in my life and asking for them back. With more gratitude than reticence, I now embrace my custodial responsibility.

Mike Arntfield, a University of Western Ontario professor and former police officer, was already working on a book about multiple serial killers in the London, Ontario, area when he heard about the discovery of detective Dennis Alsop's notes. The information found in that box provided a starting point for Arntfield's own civilian investigation and subsequent documentary, *To Catch a Killer*, which aired on the Oprah Winfrey Network in 2015.

Once again, my family was pulled into the hopeful prospect of answers. Willingly, my mom and her brothers participated in the investigation and production of the show. It was a grueling time for them. After it was over and my mom was debriefed, she previewed the episode and immediately called me up.

"I hate him," she said about Arntfield. "I want to kill him." My mom really wanted me to participate in her anger. She desperately wanted us to be mad together. She didn't know what else to do.

The theories expressed by Arntfield about what happened to Lynda were worse than any we'd imagined. And by this time, we had almost fifty years of imagining some pretty terrible shit.

"Just watch it," my mom said.

"I can't," I said.

I see what it's doing to you. I'm trying my hardest not to think about this anymore.

Mom hated the sensationalism. She hated Mike Arntfield's attitude. Mostly though, she hated his speculations.

I was afraid my mom was going to crash. "Have you thought about going back to therapy, Mom?" I said.

Arntfield's book and TV show did prompt a revival of Lynda's case by the Ontario Police. We were grateful for that. In the end, none of Arntfield's findings were confirmed, and we were back to square one. It's my theory that, in the years that followed, my mom's copious amount of fuel consumption from the Anger Gas Station contributed to her massive stroke. She now lives in a long-term care home. Like her father before her, she has aphasia and can no longer talk.

Fuel for Everyone

In Victimtown, there's only one place to get fuel. The Anger Gas Station is open twenty-four hours a day, seven days a week. We learn how to pump gas when we're kids. We watch our parents or other adults do it. We see how the different types of fuel perform, and as we grow up, we're both eager and afraid to get behind the wheel. We don't fully understand that the fuel we choose and how we use it influences our place in the world. It will either make us part of the solution or part of the problem.

Full-service pumps still exist in Victimtown. The owner is happy to chat with us as he fills our tanks. He loves his job, and he tells us, "You have every right to be furious! Someone needs to put that guy in his place."

Regular, Please

The regular fuel is called anger, and the price fluctuates. The owner charges us indiscriminately, but he tallies our bill at the end of each month. He's in cahoots with the Control Factory Boss, the Resentment Parking Lot Attendant, and the Maître D'. Together, they set the price of gas. Sometimes, for shits and giggles, they lower the price, creating long lineups. They laugh their heads off watching people get out of their cars in a frenzy and start yelling at each other as they fight to fill up.

Not satisfied with the size of their gas tank, some people bring extra containers, so they've got fuel on hand whenever they need it. These king-of-the-road type of people, they love road trips, and having to stop at the gas station every time slows them down. They tend to use a lot of fuel at home too. Angry gas is used in their kitchens, backyards, and other places. From time to time, they try to use quieter tools, but they can't seem to get much of anything done without resorting to some gas-powered device.

Other people drive distinctive vehicles with their own agendas and destinations. Each road trip requires different types and amounts of fuel. Most of our excursions are impulsive. Rarely do we plan these trips in advance. We often have no idea where we're headed when we fill up, but with an *all-in* attitude, we don't think twice. Driving furiously delivers the adrenaline rush that we crave. We get behind the wheel and we are transformed. Leaning into our power and determination, we feel our heart rates increase the faster we drive. Our blood pressure too! With sticky palms, we grip the wheel tightly and burn out. We might even flip the bird to the owner as we leave.

Some of us are taught a few safety protocols, but most of us have to figure that shit out on our own. Victimtown isn't big on rules. There are no speed limits. There are no traffic lights. In fact, there are no driving laws whatsoever. There used to be rules, but nobody followed them, and one day the town council just said, "Screw it." As a result, car crashes happen daily. The hospital here has more ambulances than any other in the world. Collateral damage is common too; it's just an odds game. Fences, houses, bike riders, and pedestrians alike are hit all the time. Sometimes with grievous injuries.

This is Victimtown.

Occasionally, drivers, hell-bent on a mission, take off without realizing there are kids in the backseat. While a few drivers don't even care, most feel remorse if something happens to them and many end up taking a hike on the trails or floating in the Sorrow Swampland.

They may seem casual and relaxed at first, but long joyrides also tend to pose problems. Those Sunday drives can quickly burn several tanks of gas. The more often we take joyrides, the more often we encounter roadblocks and mechanical problems. We have absolutely no patience for that shit. Detours drive us crazy. And they are everywhere in Victimtown. Road construction never stops. Ever.

Some people habitually fill up and then decide to postpone their trip. If the destination is depressing or we feel unequipped and afraid to make the trip, we just pull over. And we sit. The longer we sit, the more fumes we breathe in. Toxicity seeps into our bodies. Eventually, when the fuel starts to go bad, it takes on the smell of resentment. Instinctively, we drive over to the Resentment Parking Lot for a while. But the day will come when we'll have to clean out the fuel tank. We can't leave it smelling like that forever.

Something Stronger

The majority of us are content with the regular fuel. We know what we can afford and are conscious of our budget. For some people, though, the anger gas isn't enough. The more unsure of ourselves we are, the more apt we are to require something stronger.

If the regular fuel doesn't satisfy someone, they'll look for something more potent. More effective. Hate is the high-octane fuel. It's far more expensive, as it contains a particular additive. The additive is called fear. Fear serves to increase the fuel's performance by an expediential amount. It's the fuel required for drag racing, where a tank is quickly burned in one race alone. Drag racing has an extremely high mortality rate. Spectators are routinely injured or killed. We're blinded to the fact that our anger is a disguise for our fear. The more afraid we already are, the more fuel we begin to crave. The owner yells, "What are you waiting for? Let 'em have it."

Fuel Clubs

Various clubs are formed by drivers with a united mission. Meeting up regularly, they strategize and stock up on fuel. Club members covet the fear additive. Rally days are frequently planned, but they happen spur-of-the-moment as well. Tapping into their huge stores of the high-octane fuel, the clubs organize dangerous and demoralizing drag races for hours on end. Often, races don't stop until there's a ten-car pileup with multiple fatalities, spectators included.

Here in Victimtown, the scenery is pretty shitty, and a lot of the roads go around in circles. It may seem like a good idea at the time to go down this road, but in hindsight, most people realize it wasn't the best idea. It's never as satisfying as we think it will be.

Using Fuel Responsibly

Eventually, we start to question our desire to burn fuel just for the sake of driving around. Everyone is entitled to their fair share of regular fuel. It's a normal part of life to require fuel for certain tasks, and sometimes it's essential to get where we need to go. When we use anger fuel thoughtfully and responsibly, our cars run smoothly with no backfiring. It's perfectly alright to go for a short drive. When we operate our vehicle safely, show respect for other drivers and especially pedestrians, we make good use of the fuel and can return home, park our car, and truly feel better for the experience.

There are times when a drive might be a good solution. Often, a short jaunt will do the trick. There are also times when much-needed excursions are long and complicated, and that's okay too. We just don't want to be driving around in circles. Wasting gas is not cool. It's not good for us or the environment. When we avoid collateral damage and accidents, a drive can be a great motivator to accomplish big things.

As we tune in, our heart voice will tell us it's okay to feel angry. Our heart voice will encourage us to listen and really hear what our anger is saying. Anger carries some of the most critical messages. For most of us, our response to fuel up and take off is a habit we learned as kids. Awareness brings an opportunity to explore other options. Perhaps a drive is not what we really need. What other activities might ease our angst? Feeling like we need to fuel up with gas might indicate that we're running low on something else. There are many types of fuel. Gas is just one. Driving around in Victimtown exposes us to all the ramifications and implications of using anger gas and the additives. It's after we've experienced the consequences of our actions that we become open to using the cleanest, most sustainable and powerful fuel source on the planet: love. The good news is we already have a never-ending supply of love, and we can call upon it whenever we want with our heart voice.

The cleanest, most sustainable and
powerful fuel source on the planet is LOVE.

CHAPTER 12

The Sorrow Swampland

There are times when explanations, no matter
how reasonable, just don't seem to help.
—*Fred Rogers,*
Life's Journeys According to Mister Rogers

I n 2010, after I hired a private investigator to find him, I traveled to
Australia to spend time with my brother. I hadn't seen him for sev-
enteen years nor spoken to him for eight. Before I left, a lot of people
told me Australia was a dangerous place. Hearing that they have one
of the highest rates of tourist deaths every year was a tad worrisome.

Not wasting any time, my baby brother sat me down for a one-hour
lecture. "I will *not* be sending you home in a body bag," he said. "So,
listen up!"

Shit. It's true. I don't even want to know what he's going to say next.

"Do you have any wine?" I said.

"Later. This is important," he said.

Then he started with the rules:

1. Swim only in Morgan Bay, never before ten a.m. and never after four p.m. Under no circumstances do you go in any deeper than your waist, or you're shark bait. *(I won't be swimming.)*

2. Use 60 SPF ten times a day. Every day. Wear long sleeves and a hat. Stay completely out of the sun from eleven a.m. until two p.m. Every clinic and doctor's office has a kit that includes a sterile scalpel, a needle, and stitches. Their motto is, "When in doubt, cut it out." Routinely, they cut on first sight 'cause it's usually skin cancer. *(Ouch.)*

3. Without fail, look before you place your feet when you're walking. Watch every single step. Never walk on the grass. Always stay in the middle of the path. Deadly snakes are everywhere. *(Won't be walking much either.)*

4. Inspect the inside of your shoes before you put your feet in them. Without fail. It's where scorpions hide. *(Flip flops it is.)*

5. Back to the hat. Wear one with a sturdy brim along with your sunnies (sunglasses). Magpies track humans and peck out their eyes. *(Seriously?)*

6. Give the kangaroos a very wide berth. They're wild and dangerous. That cute little claw on their tiny arms can splay a person open from neck to navel in one very quick swipe. *(Got it. Lots of stitches.)*

7. Never touch a fish unless you ask me first. One touch of the wrong fish could have you hospitalized for months, feeling as if your entire body is on fire. People usually survive, but they wish every day, for months, to die. *(Okay. . . .)*

8. NEVER, ever, walk out on the rocks by the ocean. You could get swept away and drown.

After the last rule, I said, "Really? What if I watch the waves for an hour, and they never touch the spot on the rocks where I want to go stand. How about then?"

"Absolutely not," he said.

"Why not?" I asked.

"There's no way to predict when it might happen. You could watch that exact spot twenty-four hours a day for months on end, and the waves would never hit it," he explained. "Then one day it does. A massive wave comes out of nowhere. I'm talking Indian Ocean massive, like you can't even imagine. It crashes over the very spot on the rock where you were having a nice time and thought you were safe.

"First it smashes you down, knocking you unconscious, and then it sucks you back into the ocean where it throws you around and beats on you mercilessly. If you manage to regain consciousness and then somehow figure out which way to swim to come up for air, you're so far away you have no idea where you are or how you'll ever get back to shore. Most likely, though, you drown before you see daylight again," he said. "Oh, and be glad that I don't live in croc territory. That's a whole 'nother ball game."

Sorry I asked.

In life, we don't always stay away from the rocks. Sometimes it's fun or adventurous to check out what's there, just for a minute or two. Sometimes we're led out onto the rocks by someone else. Sometimes we're not even aware that we're on a rock. And sometimes, we find ourselves in a situation where there's no choice but to be on a rock for a little bit.

Approaching the Swampland

While I'm happy to report I also survived my trip to Australia, its dangers reminded me of another dangerous place: the Sorrow Swampland. As we approach the swampland, the present moment seems to disappear. Our bodies are there, but our minds and our hearts are not. Feeling both light and heavy at the same time, we are entranced by the blanket of mist that seeps up from the swamp. So very pretty, the mist leaves us mesmerized by its exquisite swirling and evocative dance until we lose all concept of time.

Well-worn paths lead to the swamp from all the places in Victimtown. People arrive of their own volition looking for a rest after an exhausting hike on the Denial Trails. A forced leave of absence from the factory due to poor performance often leads us to the swampland. When a meal at the Guilt & Shame Café leaves us feeling sick, we often decide to walk over here. The folks who don't walk or drive here on their own, well, those are the ones who get catapulted right into the middle of the swamp. Literally out of nowhere. They have the toughest time of everyone.

Cobblestone pathways crisscross each other as they meander around the perimeter of the swamp. More than enough comfortable benches are placed at perfect intervals along the paths, close enough to make eye contact with whoever's sitting on the next bench but far enough apart to provide a measure of privacy and to muffle the noises from the factory and the roads. The only sounds we hear are birds chirping, the breeze blowing, and the faint whispering messages carried by the mist.

Worry and Rumination Rafts

Two types of rafts are available for use along the shoreline of the Sorrow Swampland. Worry rafts are tied up at one end of the swamp, and the Rumination rafts are not far away on the other side. Much like the raft Huckleberry Finn used, each raft comes with long poles to maneuver it. Whether we choose a Worry or Rumination raft, any movement is tough slogging. The swamp is thick with muck, so it's almost impossible to make any progress. Mostly, we just float in one place. There's nowhere to go anyway. Sitting cross-legged or with our feet dangling in the water, we gaze into the mist and either make up a new story or remember an old one.

While a lot of people savor a solo journey on their raft, others like to share their stories. We call it a *flotilla* when rafts hang out together in the middle of the swamp. There's a fellowship to the support that each raft offers with words of confirmation and understanding. Rafts can be rented by the hour, the day, or even by the month or year. No discounts are given for long-term rentals. In fact, it's quite the opposite. The longer we use the rafts, the more our feelings rage out of control—hate, anger, shame, and fear top the list. The mist is proficient at swirling these emotions together, creating a thick cloud of anxiety that's capable of choking us.

Swamp Swimming

In between the raft rental locations lies a smaller area of the swamp where the reeds along the shoreline have been cleared, creating an area that beckons us to swim. If we succumb to the voice and are drawn into the swamp, we'll find the water warm and soothing at first. It seems to welcome us. Imagining we are safe, we find comfort as we float gently on our backs or swim slowly along the surface. The further we swim, the louder we hear the sweet song that promises to assuage our grief. A benevolent calling, the notes seep deep into our pores. The whispers become songs carrying words like, "It's just not possible to ever overcome this" and "Your life is hopeless."

And then, "No one can hurt you here," and "Stay and be forever consoled."

For as long as we remain on the surface, floating or swimming, what lies at the bottom cannot reach us. However, greater dangers loom without the protection of our raft. Deeper down, the swamp contains toxins that are detrimental to our health. Only strong swimmers have the stamina to stay on the surface, for the songs, when we listen intently or for too long, can put us into a trance and we will start to sink. With our hearts already bearing too much weight to keep us afloat, the lyrics use the power of fear to drag us to the bottom of the swamp. There, we'll meet the source of the mist messages, the singer of the songs: the Swamp Monster. If we get too close, we'll be ensnared by his grip, as the Monster has an insatiable need for new friends. He sings loudly, making us feel that our tragedy is insurmountable and that we'll never be able to move on. "Your pain will never end," he tells us. He sings and sings in his attempts to keep us too afraid to leave. More than anything, he wants us close to him, forever stuck in the swamp.

Rogue Waves

Tragic events happen. And shitstorms of epic proportions. Out of nowhere, they hit us like a rogue wave. Almost never can we predict when these occur. Shocked and undeserving, we might find ourselves suddenly sinking to the bottom of the swamp.

Newcomers will find the swamp very misleading; it's hard to fathom just how deep and thick it really is. Or what exists down there. Unaware of the risks, many a swimmer will dive down intentionally with hopeful expectation that the closer they get to the lyrics, the sooner their pain will be gone. This is sheer folly of course, because doing so will force them to succumb to the Monster that lives at the bottom. With shattered and heavy hearts, we are no match for its power of forceful fear, as it pulls us into the thick muck of grief where toxicity levels are dangerously high. Impacting our health in every way imaginable, the swamp makes us susceptible to life-long infections when we remain here.

The Monster loves to watch as the muck holds us and begins to consume us. We sing along and relive all of our past hurts, the wrongdoings against us, and the undeserved tragedies that befell us. It's a playlist that confines us. The Monster also controls the mist around the rafts. With a warped sense of humor, he fabricates specific and personal messages for everyone. More than anything, he wants to draw us into the water, lure us to the bottom, and make us keep him company forever.

There is no peace when we're near the Sorrow Swampland. Whether we're on a raft worrying about the future or ruminating about the past, whether we're swimming or sinking into its depths, our breath labors and our hearts hurt. Some people can't seem to stay away from these songs. The fear instilled by the Monster's lyrics makes us believe the swamp is where we need to be, and before we know it, we're hanging out here all the GD time.

Many of us know how it feels to be stuck deep in the muck of the swamp. Working through grief is one of the hardest things that humans experience. One of life's greatest feats is to make our way out of the swamp, particularly if we end up at the bottom. The Monster tells us that leaving the swamp equates to dismissing or forgetting entirely what we've lost. That's just not true. He also says that mourning forever is more important than caring for ourselves. Again, he's a liar. When we're grieving deeply, loving ourselves is more essential than ever to finding a way out of the swamp, and we don't have to do it alone. There are other rafts—life rafts—in the form of friends, loved ones, therapists, doctors, spiritual healers, or counselors, many of whom are ready and waiting for us with life-saving equipment. And if there's nobody around when we need help coming up for air and swimming to shore, we can turn to our heart voice for all the strength required.

At The Place, I came to understand the hows and whys around the significance of childhood traumas and the healing benefits of forgiveness. I didn't want to at first, but I did end up doing the (hard) work to unpack and reconcile both my early years and my abusive marriage. It was the gnarliest thing I've ever done, and I was so sure that would fix me. In fact, I was counting on it. But it wasn't enough. Because months later, I was still yearning. It was the yearning that brought back the doom and landed me once again in the Sorrow Swampland. I could hear the Monster singing; it was a song stuck in my head that I couldn't shake. I even heard him singing in my dreams: "Your life suuuuucks."

Sunrays

Even when our heart is broken, and perhaps *especially* when our heart is broken, our heart's still there to support us. Always. Our heart voice has the power to pull us back to the present moment where our past experiences are over. Our heart voice reminds us that we survived. Whether triumphantly, adequately, or just barely, we successfully endured all the hurts, wrongdoings, and tragedies. We're still here. Like a ray of sunshine, our heart voice can shed a different light, a light that cuts through the mist to reveal a way out and cheer us along by letting us know that everything will be okay and all we need to do is trust and relax. Our heart voice reminds us that, even though you've taken a shit-kicking, you're always in the right place at the right time doing the right thing.

You're always in the right place at the
right time doing the right thing.

Unable to see a single ray of sunshine, the Monster had a tight grip on my nana. She was stuck in the swamp for a long time. Only after Bampa had a stroke and people sent immense sunshine her way was she able to get out of the swamp to care for him. Every human will experience grief at some point in their lives. Most of us will land in the swamp when tragedy strikes.

While I'm not an expert in this most difficult emotion, I do know that grief lives in the Sorrow Swampland. And I do know that some people need to be here longer than others. And that people sink to varying degrees, even in response to similar experiences. When we're able to set judgment aside, of others or ourselves, the swamp can provide short-term solace. Our time at the swamp and our relationship with the Monster are ours and ours alone.

We all come here from time to time. The difference is what we do when we arrive. If we stay too long, the swamp will start to smell. The choice is ours. We can walk along the outskirts of the swamp and gaze into its depths. We can invite the mist to envelop and comfort us while we enjoy warm memories and stroll along. We can even relax on one of the comfy benches and dream about all that we desire and yearn for. Feeling calm and comforted, we can be grateful for this place. The swamp looks beautiful from the safety of our seat. The sun is shining, and our heart voice tells us when it's time to move along. The swamp has two purposes: It can provide healing, or it can conjure up our demise.

CHAPTER 13

The Meditation Meadow

Instead of thinking out of the box,
get rid of the box.
—*Deepak Chopra*

At the end of September, after I moved into my grandparents' house, I was the *new girl* at school. Still a little shaky from adjusting to Lynda's bedroom and still very much afraid of getting snatched, I was on high alert. It was before recess on my first day and I hadn't yet met any of my fourth-grade classmates when it happened.

Maybe I was bored, I might've been tired, or just in a daze. I don't remember. But I do know that it would never have happened if my mouth hadn't been open while I was sitting in math class. Now, I can't imagine my mouth was completely wide open, but obviously there was more than enough space between my lips. Something flew in. I shit you not. And it was buzzing around in there, banging the insides of my cheeks and the roof of my mouth.

Quick, close your mouth. If anyone sees a fly come flying out of your mouth, you'll be known as the "fly girl" and your life at this new school will be over. Forever.

It took all of my concentration to sit still. As the fly valiantly searched for an exit, my eyes betrayed me and got bigger and bigger as I mentally gauged whether the kid sitting in the desk next to me would be able to hear the buzzing, because in my head it was super loud.

What if it flies out your nose? Plug your nose.

No, don't plug your nose; some kid will ask what you're doing.

Feeling like I was about to scream, I took a deep breath (through my nose) and closed my eyes. Another breath. Slowly. And another. I started to calm down.

And then it came to me. I knew what I had to do. It was my only option. With focus and determination, I opened my eyes, gripped the sides of my chair with both hands, and took one more deep breath, as I counted to three. And then, with pursed lips, I swallowed. I swallowed hard. But it didn't go all the way down. Now it was stuck in my throat. And it was still buzzing.

Water! I need water.

I thought about putting my hand up to ask if I could go get a drink from the fountain in the hall, but I knew opening my mouth just yet was too risky. So, conjuring up as much saliva as I could, I swallowed again. And again. I kept swallowing until I couldn't feel that fly flying around inside me anymore.

The Meditation Meadow is a sacred place. It existed long before the Ego Arena was built, and it will prevail in Victimtown as a safe haven forever. Located on the far edge of town, the Meditation Meadow is a wonderous place, in every sense of the word. An invisible perimeter shield muffles all the obnoxious town voices to provide a reprieve from their shitty messages, making this place the only possibility for a little serenity in the midst of Victimtown chaos.

The Meditation Meadow is also magic. It can be both imaginary and real. Sometimes it's hard to tell the difference. But it doesn't matter. What we see when we're here is whatever gives us solace. Our hearts determine all the details of the meadow. Some people see an ocean or a vista of rolling hills or a dense forest. Some people see rocky mountains or a vast desert. Regardless of our vision, the same sense of calm is available for everyone who comes here.

The soil, the sun, and the air are all calibrated to provide an abundance of the nutrients required for our hearts to thrive. The entire populace of Victimtown has a heart problem, and the meadow holds immense healing powers that can prevent us from ending up at the Epiphany Hospital.

Occasionally, the Boss and her cronies do show up here, but there's something about the environment that makes them uneasy. They seem to sense that, here in the meadow, they've got competition to garner our attention. Eventually, the town voices realize that their time is better spent at all the other places in Victimtown where their voices are amplified and people listen willingly.

Although our time here can be either sedentary or active, it's always a solo experience. That's not to say that there aren't other people here, because there are, but everyone keeps to themselves. The sounds of nature are pretty much all we hear in the meadow. Rustling leaves, birdsong, trickling brooks, whistling winds, or crashing waves. Quite literally, it's the only place in Victimtown that provides any measure of peace.

In our own time, and for our own reasons, some of us discover this sanctuary while we're in Victimtown. Without the intrusive and abusive town voices, something extraordinary occurs here: Our heart voice shows up. It might not happen right away, but our heart voice has been begging to be heard, and there are no better conditions on earth for it to make itself known.

It's also here, in the quiet of the Meditation Meadow, where many people first feel the desire to leave Victimtown. The more time we spend here, the better, because in due course, we will undoubtedly hear what our hearts have been patiently waiting to tell us. Plans to leave can be thoughtfully formulated. There is a playlist available here that will guide and support us on our road trip to Freedomville.

Beauty exists everywhere in the meadow. This beauty propels us to imagine everything that's possible. We can see and feel what our lives could look like. Hope is in the air, and we breathe it in deeply. Respair lies under every rock.

Returning to this meadow as often as we need, we have no better place to gather the courage to begin our journey out. The meadow can also provide the strength needed to continue when the going gets tough. Solutions sometimes appear seemingly out of thin air in the meadow, which can be a huge relief when we run into roadblocks trying to leave town.

Not everyone chooses to come here, though. The Dirtbags tell hikers that the meadow is a myth. The Monster makes up stories about crazy-ass dangers in the meadow, and while the Boss is yelling at us to get back to our jobs, the Maître D' informs us that we don't qualify to be here anyway. Some of us are shown the way here by a friend who's come to visit us from Freedomville. It's also possible that we stumble upon the meadow by accident.

There are paths out of Victimtown that can only be accessed from this meadow. The number of visits here and length of time it takes for us to find these exit routes are different for all of us. While we're gearing up to leave town, the benefits and positive effects of the meadow follow us. With each subsequent return to our jobs at the Control Factory or to any of the other places in Victimtown, we start to become a bit skeptical about what the town voices have to say, and we begin to comprehend that as long as we're still in town, we're dangerously susceptible to their shitty, violent, and never-ending messages.

Everything our hearts imagine for ourselves while we're in the meadow can become our reality.

Everything.

CHAPTER 14

The Epiphany Hospital

Anyone can be a fool and do things which are wrong,
but fools find out when it's too late
that they don't live so long.
—*Jiminy Cricket,* Pinocchio *(1940)*

In the sixth grade, I made the track team. I was the third runner on a 4 x 100 relay team. It's the weakest runner's position, but I didn't care. We had a shot at a medal because the other girls were top-notch athletes. The county finals were held at the high school with a professional track and proper stands for spectators. It felt like the big leagues! Multiple events were going on simultaneously: the long jump, high jump, and all kinds of races. This one race would determine whether we advanced to the provincial championships.

My parents said they'd be there to cheer us on. When it was time for our race, I couldn't find them anywhere.

Where are they? Why aren't they here?

I walked to my position halfway around the track.

I'm sure they're here somewhere; I just don't see them.

I scanned the stands again. I even looked beyond the stands at the stragglers walking from the parking lot.

I can't believe it. They forgot.

The starting gun fired, and as I watched the first runners take off, I got a funny feeling in the pit of my stomach.

Something's wrong.

The niggly feeling of dread got stronger. I shoved it down, but there was a lump in my stomach. Runner number two now had the baton. I started running before she reached me. I grabbed the baton and took off.

Whatever you do, Liz, do not drop this baton.

My focus shifted from hanging onto the baton to outrunning the dread in my gut, and I had never run faster. I passed the baton to our last runner, slowed to a jog, and checked the stands. My family wasn't there.

What's happened?

Panic bubbled up in my throat, and I knew without knowing how I knew, that I had to go home. Immediately. Without stopping my jog, I veered off toward the parking lot.

"Where are you going? The race isn't over!" my coach yelled.

"Gotta go home," I shouted back.

Those four blocks took forever. I rounded the last corner and saw five police cars lined up, one behind the other, five red domes in a row in my circular driveway. It stopped me in my tracks. With my hands on my knees, I hung my head and caught my breath. Then I looked long and hard at the police cars. It wasn't unusual to see one there. But not five. I knew because I felt it. Lynda had been found.

It took several days for the police to confirm Lynda's identity. Of course, I was sad. We were all heartbroken, but I felt something else too. Relief.

Finally. It's all behind us. Thank God.

I felt guilty and ashamed for feeling relieved. I couldn't help it.

How can I be happy that my favorite aunt is dead?

It wasn't a giddy, fun kind of happy. It was more of a resigned kind of happy. Nonetheless, it felt so very wrong, and it was not something I wanted, but there it was. I think it was more that I was happy about what all this meant, that it wouldn't be hanging over our lives anymore. That the police would stop coming to our house. That all the questions would be answered. That they'd catch the killer and I wouldn't have to be afraid anymore. That my mom would love me now. That there wouldn't be any more newspaper articles. That all of it—this entire, huge never-ending shitstorm—was finally behind us.

But it wasn't. And it's still not. That's the thing about life. Nothing is over until we learn whatever lesson was meant for us. It won't end until we heal. It can't. And after that, a new lesson will arrive (aka, shit happens). Nobody has the power to stop it. It's the way the universe works.

Entering the Epiphany Hospital

Located on the edge of Victimtown is the Epiphany Hospital. It's a world-class teaching facility and one of the largest and most renowned medical facilities on earth. This hospital attracts the very best healthcare providers. Some of them live in town, while others commute daily from nearby Freedomville to offer their services to the people who need them most.

Although quite basic and institutional in its décor, this hospital boasts all the best equipment and technology. Patients receive immediate care with unlimited access to diagnostic tests and treatments. With specialty practitioners in all departments, the Epiphany Hospital is equipped to handle every physical and mental condition you can imagine. If you need acute medical care, you really wanna be at Epiphany, because it's here that the world's best opportunities and outcomes are offered.

Ambulances bring a constant stream of patients from the Control Factory, the Guilt & Shame Café, and the Resentment Parking Lot. The volume of car accidents can be predicted by gas and additive sales at the Anger Gas Station. The Freedomville Search and Rescue teams are frequently called to save people who've been injured on the Denial Trails. People also walk in on their own from the Sorrow Swampland.

Everyone arriving by ambulance is in some state of shock. Ample time is devoted to all incoming patients to explain the extent of services available and to answer questions. Arriving here is a wake-up call from the universe, but not everyone's ready for it. The staff is used to people refusing treatment, although there's no rhyme or reason as to which ones choose to leave. But there is one clue: Most patients who refuse treatment were seen in close conversation with a town volunteer while waiting to see the doctor. The doctors know from experience that their time is best spent with the patients who see their chance at leaving Victimtown. The others are given a brochure and released.

Young and old, from all walks of life, the only thing people here have in common are their issues. In the various departments, however, they all find solace in the fact that they are not alone. Everyone is surprised to learn just how many others have similar problems. There's an atmosphere of respair at Epiphany Hospital. And it describes perfectly the vibe that's found here.

The town council (the Boss and all of her cohorts) depend on the population of Victimtown for the economy to run the way they like it. It doesn't help their cause when people leave. So, they all volunteer to visit patients every day. The Boss makes sure they all take this responsibility seriously and that time is spent with everyone individually. Patients who enjoy listening to the same volunteers tend to gravitate to each other.

The town council volunteers love to tell stories and give advice. They talk and talk and talk. Here's what some of them might say:

> The Boss: "You don't have time for this shit. You're losing money lying here. Get your ass back to work."
> The Maître D': "You brought this on yourself. You're pathetic, weak, and deficient."

The Resentment Parking Lot Attendant: "You got your father's genes. It's all his fault" or "Your body has betrayed you."

The Gas Station Manager: "This is so unfair. Someone should pay for this!"

The Swampland Monster: "You're probably gonna die. Even if you live, you'll never be the same."

The Dirtbag: "Don't worry, this is just a freak thing. It won't happen again" or "The doctors don't know what they're talking about."

In April 2021, Jonathan Frostick, a forty-five-year-old Brit, posted this on LinkedIn:

"So I had a heart attack . . .

This is not how I planned my Sunday. It was pretty standard up to 4:00 p.m. Morning coffee, a trip to the local country park, a shopping trip, and late lunch.

I sat down at my desk at 4:00 p.m. to prep for this week's work. And then I couldn't really breathe. My chest felt constrained. I had what I can only describe as surges in my left arm, my neck, my ears were popping.

I didn't get a flash of light, my life raced through my mind. Instead I had:

1. Fuck I needed to meet with my manager tomorrow; this isn't convenient.

2. How do I secure the funding for X (work stuff)?

3. Shit I haven't updated my will.

4. I hope my wife doesn't find me dead.

I got to the bedroom so I could lie down and got the attention of my wife who phoned 999.

I've since made the following decisions whilst I've laid here, on the basis I don't die:

1. I'm not spending all day on Zoom anymore.

2. I'm restructuring my approach to work.

3. I'm really not going to be putting up with any s#%t at work ever again—life literally is too short.

4. I'm losing 15 kg.

5. I want every day to count for something at work, else I'm changing my role.

6. I want to spend more time with my family.

And that, so far, is what near death has taught me."[1]

I wasn't surprised to see that, as of this writing, his post has 297,857 likes and 15,479 comments. Heart attacks and accidents bring people to the hospital daily. Most are in disbelief upon arrival, even the ones who've been warned. Nobody expects to end up in this place. Not really. A few may have an inkling that it's a possibility, but they don't really think it will happen. Not to them, anyway.

For some of us it takes a stay at this hospital to hear our heart voice for the first time. It may start by saying, "Could it be time to make some changes?" or "Maybe money at the expense of stress isn't worth it," and "It's never too late."

There are three ways to leave the Epiphany Hospital:

1. We can exit through the door we came in and return to Victimtown.

2. We can decide to begin our healing journey and arrange whatever support we need to help us find our way to a better place.

3. We die and our time on earth ends.

There's a chance for a big change of heart while recovering here. If we survive, our next steps will take some planning. Where will we go? We hear rumblings about a place called Freedomville . . . A place that feels far away and yet familiar in a déjà vu kinda way.

No doubt there's comfort in returning to our life in Victimtown, entrenched in our established routines and our relationships. A voice says, "Better the devil that you know." Even if things are shitty, we won't have too many surprises. Well, other than perhaps an inconvenient trip to the hospital. But we'll soon forget about that. With their conniving messages, the volunteers urge us to discount, ignore, or forget all the facts and events that are either painful to face or scare the shit out of us.

I'd hazard a guess that a decent portion of those fifteen thousand people who commented on Jonathan Frostick's post with empathic words of understanding were still thinking there must be some specific reason it happened to him that *didn't apply* to them. "He must've been really out of shape. He probably had bad genes, too."

When we hear things like that in our head, now we can smell the bullshit of that line of reasoning.

Our Chances at the Epiphany Hospital

What are my chances? How many chances do I get? Is this my last chance? Please, I want another chance! These words echo in the halls at the Epiphany Hospital daily. If we've been here before, we might start to question what the town council volunteers keep telling us. If we can decide that we're just not up for visitors anymore, we'll be free to hear more from our heart voice in the quiet. Our hearts have all the answers.

Here's what I believe. Our hearts extend to us an infinite number of chances. Unfortunately, they just aren't all in this lifetime. None of us ever know how many chances we've got left on this go-round. It makes sense to me, then, that it's best to take advantage of the chance in hand as soon as we become aware of it.

> Our hearts extend to us an infinite
> number of chances. Unfortunately,
> they just aren't all in this lifetime.

The doctors at this hospital will call a spade a spade. A comprehensive and complete range of diagnostic services are provided so everyone has the most accurate information possible about their current condition. Sometimes the news is not good. It's hard to accept that a long hike won't change it or make it go away, but now we know in our hearts the truth of that. It's time to figure out our shit best way we can. Lean into respair, become hopeful, and I promise that your heart won't let you down.

And for those interested in doing the work, support departments are located on the top floor where you'll find psychologists, psychotherapy, physiotherapy, and hypnotherapy. Nutritionists, infection control, and counseling, too. There's even a finance department and a chaplain. Personal trainers, life coaches, and meditation circles also exist. Epiphany offers intuitive healers and spiritual awakeners, art therapy and nature therapy, anger release therapy, addiction treatments, and support for family members. Options abound for awareness and support here. Epiphany offers us a chance to stay at the hospital if we need any of these services urgently.

We decide what playlist we want to listen to. If we're already yearning for something more, returning to Victimtown will only intensify our unfulfillment and unhappiness. Although it may seem easier in the short term, the longer we remain in Victimtown, the more likely we are to end up in the Epiphany Hospital. Hospital stays can be either enlightening or senseless. Our hearts are so much stronger than we realize. Every experience, every shitty thing that has happened to us, can eventually be healed. I wasn't aware of it at the time, but while I was at The Place, my heart voice was getting stronger.

The Epiphany Hospital offers its patients one of the easiest ways out. After all, they've been through a lot, and they survived. A sky-walk connects the hospital directly to Freedomville. As we traverse it, Victimtown can be viewed from a distance, and the town voices become less audible the closer we get to Freedomville. Inspired to lead a different life, most of us are excited and scared in equal measures.

That's 100 percent normal.

Not everyone leaves Victimtown from the hospital. In fact, most of us take the slow road out. The entire population of Victimtown has heart problems. The yearning seeds start to sprout while we're eating at the café or floating in the swamp or while we're huffing and puffing to catch our breath as we hike the steep trails and we start to think, "There's GOTTA be more to life."

It's inevitable. We'll all land in Victimtown at some point or another to heal or learn another lesson because life continues to throw curveballs. But mostly because, to varying degrees, every single one of us is a victim of our childhood.

To varying degrees, every single one
of us is a victim of our childhood.

PART 3

Leaving Victimtown

CHAPTER 15

The Shitty Life Circle

What a wonderful life I've had!
I only wish I'd realized it sooner.
—*Sidonie-Gabrielle Colette*

N one of us planned it. Nobody wished for it. "When I grow up, I want to be a victim," said nobody. Ever. It happened little by little, bit by bit, as things have a way of doing when we're just trying to hang on. We didn't even know it, but we'd landed in Victimtown. And then we got stuck there because we believed the town voices. We continued to listen to their playlists and navigated new shitstorms the same way we always did—with fear. We leaned into our familiar and trusted childhood coping mechanisms, and we armored up to protect ourselves or to find comfort and solace. Here's what it looks like:

THE SHITTY LIFE CIRCLE

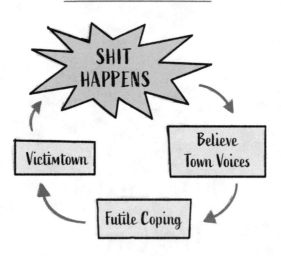

I made this up in an effort to explain my life. The Shitty Life Circle. I mean, my life hasn't been all bad. But whenever shit happened, this was the circle I was on. For over fifty years, I kept going around and around. I didn't know it until I knew it. When I first conceived this, a town voice told me I was a bit slow. Fifty years is kind of a long time to be doing laps around this circle. But now that I understand how it works, I'm coming to terms with it. And—spoiler alert—when I learned how to disrupt the Shitty Life Circle, well, that's when everything shifted.

As we grew up, we armored up. We had no choice. We ventured out into the world on our own, and we had to protect our hearts. Every time something went wrong, our interpretation justified our shitty childhood beliefs and provided another perfect example of what the town voices told us to expect. In response, we added a little bit more weight or another piece of armor. It was for our own safety and protection. Better to be safe than sorry, right?

Don't Feel Bad

It's not just you. Or me. Every human on earth has experienced this Shitty Life Circle. And we all rationalize it in our own way.

The tendency to minimize our traumas is common, especially if they weren't the worst thing imaginable. A lot of us downplay our struggles. We don't want to admit how bad it really was, let alone share it with other people. It starts with the little things on the surface of our everyday life. Someone asks you, "Hey, how are you?" You automatically reply, "I'm great, thanks, how are you?" But the truth is maybe you're not feeling great right now. Maybe you're feeling exhausted or worried or stressed, but you don't even want to think about it yourself, let alone talk about it. Or, if you consider answering with the truth, a town voice shows up and tells you that, surely, this person doesn't really want to hear it. The truth is, a lot of us *don't* want to know all about other people's problems. Not because we don't care, but because we're unsure how to respond. We're afraid of saying or doing the wrong thing. When we can't admit and share the small issues that are less-than-great, it becomes more challenging to address the bigger traumatic stuff that happened in our past. So, we don't. When we can't speak our truth, we can't get off this circle, and we stay in Victimtown.

Some of us tend to overemphasize the severity of other people's problems because then, by comparison, our problems are lessened and we feel better. I'm going to be honest with you: This is cheating. We can always find someone who had a worse experience than us. But that doesn't invalidate what we went through. We can also always find someone whose problems are not as bad as ours. It's not helpful, or relevant, to compare our childhood experiences, or any shit that happens in our present lives, with anyone else. Playing the blame game also keeps us going around this circle. Even though it may help us feel better momentarily, blaming is an ineffective way to disrupt this cycle.

On occasion, we even completely dismiss our response to traumas because we don't feel *entitled* to our reaction. We don't believe that it's okay or acceptable to feel hurt. We judge and quantify what feelings we're entitled to have. Not feeling our feelings also keeps us on the Shitty Life Circle.

We were born full of love with strong, open hearts brimming with innate wisdom. We were along for the ride and then shit happened. Doing the best we could, we made up stories about what it all meant that resulted in some pretty shitty beliefs. Then, to protect ourselves and make sure it never happened again, we got creative and adopted new behaviors and coping mechanisms, all of which kept us on this Shitty Life Circle.

It doesn't take that much shit to cause us to lose our way and begin to follow the road of fear. In fact, it takes much less than you might think. So, if you're saying to yourself, "My childhood wasn't that bad," if you're struggling to find the connection between your past and your current unhappy life, I invite you to reflect and to dig a little. Get introspective. Then dig a little more. Journal. Talk to a therapist and set the intention to make the connection. I promise you, the connection is there, and you need to find it because it's what's keeping you on the Shitty Life Circle. Your subconscious can start working on it right now. All you have to do is ask.

Through no fault of our own, we became inadvertent victims of our childhoods.

That's how we arrived in Victimtown.

Then we ended up on the Shitty Life Circle.

And that's how we got stuck in Victimtown.

Looping 'round the Shitty Life Circle
keeps us stuck in Victimtown.

Emily Maroutian, an author and poet born in Armenia, said it well: "You did the best you could with the knowledge you had in that moment. It's easier to look back at an event and see a better choice or pathway because we already learned from our experience. Hindsight happens after the lesson, so we can't condemn ourselves for not knowing the lesson before we learned it."[1]

Everything that happened to us in our childhood made us who we are today. We are, as individuals, a sum of what we've been through. Our unique adverse childhood experiences, our stories, our new beliefs, and all of our creative coping mechanisms led us to be exactly who and where we are today. And who and where we are today is exactly who and where we were meant to be—a humble human who realizes where they've been hanging out in Victimtown and understands how they got there. Now it's time to blow this popsicle stand.

CHAPTER 16

Exit Stage Left

You're braver than you believe,
stronger than you seem,
and smarter than you think.
—*Christopher Robin*, Winnie-the-Pooh, *A.A. Milne*

The day we admit we're stuck in Victimtown is a good day and a bad day. Major turning points in life are typically like that. It takes a certain level of pain to get our attention. We can't change our past. What we can do is start from wherever we are right now. Getting real about our current situation is half the battle. It makes no difference how long you've been in Victimtown. You're ready when you're ready. The Hanna-Barbera cartoon character Snagglepuss said, "Exit, stage left!" It's that simple. Well, sort of. Like our arrivals, our exits from Victimtown can also be messy and a bit convoluted. Everyone takes a different path. And that's okay. There are lots of routes to explore, and we get better at navigating our quintessential journey with practice. What matters is that we've decided to pursue more peace, love, freedom, or joy. That's important, huge even. Because, if we stay in Victimtown, all we'll get is chaos, apathy, enslavement, and depression (aka, shit).

Our childhood beliefs resulted in coping mechanisms that cut us off from the only muscle capable to defeat the town voices—our hearts. Our hearts are designed to gain strength through our suffering, to accumulate knowledge from our most painful experiences. These *heartfelt* insights are precisely what will get us out of Victimtown. Trust me, you have it in you—you just need to access your own heartfelt wisdom.

Planning and preparation are required for all road trips, and what's more important than an expedition to find fulfillment and happiness? It's essential to know who's on our team and who isn't. Our lives are not about other people. Our lives belong to us. The question to ask is, "How much do we care about ourselves?"

Waiting for someone to save us is just an excuse to continue to hang out in Victimtown. Expecting others to do for us what we haven't yet done for ourselves isn't realistic or fair. It's not fair to them, but mostly it's not fair to us. Other people can help us, sure. They can show us the way and provide support, but we can never rely on others entirely. And we don't have to. Our heart voice knows the way out.

Our heart voice knows the way out of Victimtown.

Roadblocks

Surprisingly, our brains aren't always working in our best interest. Our brains are biased to reinforce the negative beliefs formed in our childhoods. We all want to be right. Plus, it's in our DNA to do that. Our brains are hardwired to interpret new experiences in a way that is consistent with whatever we already believe. Go figure. This makes it popular, understandable, and even excusable for our childhood coping mechanisms to grow up with us and morph into adult behaviors.

Whether we're ensconced in Victimtown or actively searching for a way out, we're predisposed to look for and to allocate a weighty meaning to all the experiences that justify how we already feel and what we already believe. We deliberately seek out evidence that proves our beliefs are correct and true. Known as confirmation bias, it's a natural tendency for almost all of us. And the town voices jump all over this and hammer it in.

Sometimes, we even distort information so that it feels more comfortable and familiar. We always get to choose what things mean. Because we feel better when things make sense and jive with our previous experiences and current (shitty) beliefs, we're inclined to assign meanings to ongoing events that support what we figured out in childhood. What's more, many of us habitually diminish or entirely discount any evidence to the contrary. What? Are we dense? No. We are human.

We always get to choose what things mean.

A brain is happy when it confirms its righteousness. Much the same as when we were figuring out meanings as kids, our brains don't like any gaps. A meaning must fill every empty space. Connections must be made. However, neither the meaning nor the connection needs to be accurate or correct. They just need to exist. The path of least resistance is for us to interpret whatever shit is happening in a way that easily fits into and supports what we already believe from our childhood. The town voices reiterate and champion this perspective because their mission is to keep us afraid so that we'll stay in Victimtown. The disconnect, the seeds of our yearnings, come about because our hearts know the truth.

It's Hard to Say Goodbye

Leaving Victimtown can be bittersweet. Even after we realize that it's time to go, it can be hard to say goodbye to familiar and comfortable places. Leaving isn't easy, but it will end our pain, and surely that's worth the effort.

As we begin to plan our exit, we see that the people who can support us in the ways we need are not the ones in Victimtown. Everyone in Victimtown is there on their own accord, for their own reasons. If some of our friends have stopped there temporarily, to regroup or learn a life lesson, they'll find their own way out in their own time. They won't be the ones to kick up a fuss about us leaving. Instead, they'll bid us adieu and wish us well as they hope to join us soon in Freedomville.

Some of our pals, however, are not gonna want to be left there without us. If they've been living there for a long time, they're in tight with the town council, and they won't want to see us go. Full of anger, sorrow, or resentment, or committed to endless hikes on the trails, these folks might take desperate measures to keep us with them. We need to be prepared for that. We can't force them to come with us, and we're not gonna try—because we've quit our jobs at the factory. We must look after ourselves first and foremost. We don't have to forget them, though. The most effective way to help them is to remind them that their own heart voice knows best. And to show them how it can be done—by not letting them hold us back. We can also encourage them to spend time in the Meditation Meadow.

The decision to leave Victimtown is yours and yours alone. You don't have to wait for anyone to come with you. You don't have to stay to look after anyone either, even the people you love. And you don't need anyone's permission. This is your life, your one and only, and it's your responsibility. And it's never too late.

The decision to leave Victimtown
is yours and yours alone.

I invite you to keep an open mind about concepts that you think are unproven or scary or weird because, whenever you think that, well, that's usually the town voices doing their best to keep you from leaving.

The Shitty Life Circle can be disrupted one new choice at a time. The last thing we want is to end up in the Epiphany Hospital.

I came up with a plan. It's a plan where your heart's in control of the playlist, not the town voices. It's a plan to help you prepare and execute your own road trip to leave Victimtown. It's how you'll find Freedomville and all that you yearn for.

It's called the Heart Voice Power Plan.

So, are ya ready to flip the bird to Victimtown?

CHAPTER 17

The Heart Voice Power Plan

It doesn't take a hero to order men into battle.
It takes a hero to be one of those men
who goes into battle.
—Norman Schwarzkopf

All the strategies in the upcoming chapters are designed to strengthen your heart voice. We have a war to fight before we can even begin our journey out of Victimtown. The town voices are the enemy, and those of us who choose to engage in this battle to fight for our yearnings are the heroes. And you guessed it—your heart voice is your best weapon. It needs to be powerful.

Physically, our heart supports our entire body. All of our organs depend on it. We can be alive without brain function. We can survive without limbs. We can donate a kidney or have our appendix or gallbladder removed, but we can't survive without our heart. Its function, however, is so much more than its physical job of pumping blood. Our heart is our soul's GPS.

Each of us has a heart. We need only to put our hand on our chest and feel it beating. Our hearts are the essence of us. The physical beat of our heart exists for us to feel its vibration and be reminded that we're not alone. Our hearts also connect us to everyone and everything in the universe.

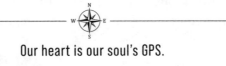

Our heart is our soul's GPS.

You may be concerned that you don't have a heart voice, or that you'll never find it, or that it's too weak, or . . . You get the picture. Before you throw in the towel, I want you to know—that voice in your head that's bringing up those concerns? That's a Victimtown voice. You'll know this, because you'll talk back to it, and it never has anything nice to say. And if you continue to listen to that voice, you'll soon begin to feel lousy.

Our heart voice has all the answers. For real. All of them. This powerful voice can support us through the worst of times, even when we question our very survival. Our hearts are all-knowing when it comes to what's for our highest and best good. Unfortunately, that will include having to endure painful feelings. Our hearts, however, can handle anything. When our heart voice rules, our intentions are based in love. And when our intentions are based in love, our hearts have the capacity to generate the endless power that's required to sustain us through even the worst shitstorms.

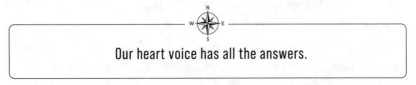

Our heart voice has all the answers.

Even with this renewed strength, there's still going to be some practical stuff that needs to happen. But the good news is our heart voice power can provide all the guidance we need for our expedition, regardless of where we've been hanging out or how long we've been stuck.

In case you're wondering what your heart voice can do, check this out. Your heart voice can:

- ♥ Defeat the town voices

- ♥ Transform your shitty beliefs from childhood

- ♥ Help you get out of Victimtown

- ♥ Enable you to adopt healthy coping mechanisms

- ♥ Sustain you when you need it most

- ♥ Encourage you to dream big

- ♥ Help you navigate any shitstorm imaginable

- ♥ Keep you from landing in Victimtown when shit happens

- ♥ Or make your stay there as short as possible

- ♥ Pave the way for you to love yourself without limits or conditions

- ♥ Inspire you to spend more time in Freedomville

You Are Your Heart

Our hearts are every bit as unique as everything else about us. To acknowledge and know our heart voice, we must first acknowledge and know ourselves. Many of us have hidden or forgotten who we are. Childhood shit can do that to us. One common belief is that our value is based, in large part, on our physical attributes. Past experiences caused us to think that if we weren't beautiful, tall, strong, athletic, or some other physical aspect, that we were not enough. Most of us are so very critical of ourselves.

Honestly, even the most beautiful people are insecure. Our value has nothing whatsoever to do with our physical appearance. Bigger boobs won't make anyone happy. I speak from experience and my ex-husband's. My heart voice would've confirmed that, but it was still too covered with armor for me to hear it. But now I want you to hear it. Loud. And. Clear.

We are all more than enough, exactly the way we are.

Presenting ourselves honestly and openly to the world is the only way we'll find our true tribe. How often do you misrepresent your interests, talents, or desires? Connecting with like-minded people can give us a feeling of belonging. If we disguise who we truly are, our associations will be based on false pretenses, and any value or meaning is diluted. It's counterproductive to be anything but our true selves, yet so many of us are afraid to show the world who we really are. Brené Brown said it well: "Our sense of belonging can never be greater than our level of self-acceptance."[1] The feeling of belonging, the love that we yearn for, is dependent on our self-acceptance.

I almost never read newspapers, and I very rarely watch the news. Hearing about all the tragedies in the world has given me anxiety my whole life, so I don't do it. But that created a different problem. At the very least I was embarrassed. Most often, though, I was ashamed to be unaware of current events, especially at cocktail parties. I used to smile and nod. I'd pretend to know what people were talking about because it was obvious that everyone else knew what was going on. Everyone, that is, except me. I prayed they wouldn't ask me anything else when my opinion was, "Yeah, I totally agree." If I was put on the spot, I'd head for the Denial Trails, especially if the person I was talking to worked at the Control Factory.

These days, I make it a bit of a joke. This is one childhood coping mechanism that I'm still working on. I think maybe my first job of cutting out articles on the porch to protect my grandparents from added grief about Lynda might've had something to do with it. At any rate, I'm now able to embrace the fact that I don't have a keen interest to discuss negative world events. It's not that I don't care; I just know that it makes me feel really shitty when I spend time reading or talking about stuff like that, so I listen more to my heart voice when it tells me not to.

My close friends and family are well aware. At my request, they've agreed to call me if something major is happening in the world, 'cause seriously, I won't have a clue. That's part of what makes me, me. What makes you, you? It's essential to figure this out, because in order to love ourselves, we need to know and understand exactly who it is we're loving.

Our hearts already love and accept us. Self-worth is the foundation, the fertile ground in which to grow our heart voice. Growing our heart voice provides and enhances this foundation of self-worth. It's not a chicken-and-egg scenario. (New quantum physics theories suggest that the chicken and egg can *both* come first.) So, before we can successfully fight the town voices, we have to believe we're worth it. And before we believe we're worth it, we must start fighting the town voices. Learning to love ourselves is our greatest achievement. The first step in that endeavor is to know ourselves thoroughly—to get real about who we are and who we are not. Our sexuality, our spirituality, and our values are all different too. Sometimes, these things evolve throughout our lives as we experience and learn new things. It's all good. What matters is that we're honest with ourselves.

Self-worth is the foundation, the fertile ground in which to grow our heart voice.

Is it human nature to compare ourselves to others, or is that a learned behavior? I think it's both. It's interesting, fun, and valuable to compare ourselves to others when we come from a place of love.

By acknowledging differences, we can communicate and validate the value of both ourselves and others. With the motivation of love, comparisons can produce amazing outcomes that are for the highest and best good for everyone involved. This is the way we were born.

The town voices, however, have a different motivation when they compare people. Those voices use comparisons to reinforce the shitty beliefs or to instill fear so they can control us. Comparisons motivated by fear lead to judgment and pit us against each other. Judgment leads to a determination and ranking of who is worth more. What hogwash! Everyone's value is inherent. We were born with it. Intrinsic human value is not something other people get to weigh in on. Period.

Here's a provocative experiment: I invite you to look at yourself in a mirror. Standing as close to the mirror as possible is preferable. Then look into your eyes. Hold the gaze, like you would with someone you're in love with. How does it feel? What thoughts come up? Relax and get a little curious. Look a little longer and probe a little deeper. See how long you can lock eyes with yourself. Who is that? Do you recognize yourself? What other feelings come up? We look into the eyes of people we love all the time. This gesture of connection communicates our feelings without words. Rarely do we take a close look at ourselves. The first time I tried it, it was weird. The town voices showed up, and I felt stupid, unsure, embarrassed, and vulnerable. I was afraid I wouldn't recognize myself. It took several attempts. And then, when I did recognize myself, I was scared the person looking back didn't (or worse, couldn't) love me in return. Over time, when I looked into my own eyes, my feelings moved along the spectrum of curiosity, acceptance, comfort, and finally love.

Intrinsic human value is not something
other people get to weigh in on.

Should you choose to accept the mission, the next level of this exercise is to say something to yourself. Something from your heart. Something like, "You're beautiful. You're smart. You can do this." Or even better, "I love you." When it comes from your heart, you'll not only hear the truth of it, but you'll also feel it in your body.

It sounds like a silly thing to do, and it'll surely be awkward if you're caught in the act, but until you've tried it, don't knock it. It's said the eyes are the "window to the soul." While I believe this, I would also add, "and to our heart and its voice."

Intuition

Our intuition resides in our heart. It's the only form of fear meant for our highest good—to keep us alive. It's also called a "gut instinct," which may lead you to think that it's a stomach thing. Although we may feel it in our gut, I think intuition's a heart thing. It's what we rely on to alert us when we're in physical danger—that is, if we're listening.

Science might explain that intuition is part of our survival instinct, something that's hard-wired into our DNA to keep us alive. There are all kinds of people, however, who couldn't explain why but knew they shouldn't do something (board the plane, get in the car, etc.), and it saved their life. That was their intuition.

I don't remember what my mom called it, but we had many discussions about it. There's been so much conjecture over the details of Lynda's death. One of the most debated points was under what circumstances she was abducted or if she willingly went along with someone. We'll never know the role that Lynda's intuition played in the way things unfolded for her, but it's possible, perhaps even likely, her intuition alerted her to danger well before her life ended. It's also possible that, as events unfolded, she recalled a previous point where her gut instinct provided warning clues that she rationalized away. This was the scenario that my mother wanted to avoid ever happening to me. It's the reason she made sure I learned at a very young age to give credence to my intuition. She didn't teach me this to make me happier or to help me find my life purpose. Rather, it was presented as a necessary skill to avoid getting snatched. It kept me on my toes. And it kept me afraid.

I can think of only one circumstance where fear is beneficial. When fear is generated by our intuition, it can keep us safe. It's a tool that can ensure our very survival. Certain groups of people, through their work or hobbies, are routinely subjected to life-threatening circumstances. When we require this level of protection, I believe it comes in the form of intuition. First responders, military personnel, arborists, miners, and extreme sport enthusiasts are some examples of people who know what I mean.

Occasionally, terrible things do happen, and no amount of gut instinct or intuition will make a difference, but the fear that's generated from our heart is sent to protect us. It's the only fear that's motivated by love. All the other fears we feel are the town voices working to control us.

Our intuition does more than alert us to imminent physical danger. Most of us have had at least one experience where we had a hunch, a sudden insight—similar to the *spidey sense* that something is wrong, but gentler and without the adrenaline. Intuition can also be subtle, like when we get a great idea or inspiration surfaces. When we have an intuitive thought, we might think at first that our brain has created it. But then, for the life of us, we can't identify exactly where the thought came from. The source is a mystery. We scour our memory for all that we've seen or heard recently, and we conclude that this thought, this great idea, did not originate from our five senses. Where, then, did it come from? It came from our heart voice.

Our intuition serves our creativity. It leads us to encounter, seemingly by chance, the resources we need for a project. It's also the source of all our inspirations and great ideas. Yep, those light-bulb moments—they all come from your heart voice! Solutions to problems that arrive in our sleep, doors opening for new opportunities, and people showing up in our lives when we need them most. None of it's random. That's our intuition at work.

We're all born with the innate ability to tap into our intuition, but we've been conditioned to expect and demand scientific evidence to prove everything. Our intuition (aka, our heart voice) puts thoughts in our heads. When our intuition tells us something that's not familiar, one of the town voices is always ready to shut it down.

We're all born with the innate ability to tap into our intuition.

We begin to override our intuition as children. This *just knowing something* is not generally supported by most cultures, and far too rarely is it taught. In turn, this makes us more reactive, because what we end up learning is not to trust ourselves. The town voices instill doubt. When we don't trust ourselves, well, that takes power away from our heart voice.

Regardless of my early knowledge that I could depend on my intuition to keep me physically safe, I didn't know how to listen to it, let alone rely on it, when I was making decisions about everything else in my life. It's easier to recognize our intuition in hindsight. Ya know, after the fact, when we're analyzing the progression of events and reliving the experience, we have that aha moment where we remember the voice in our head or the way we felt. For a split second, we knew that another path might be a better choice, but we let a town voice talk us out of it. "Right! Maybe next time I'll listen," we think. It doesn't have to be that way. We can start listening to our heart voice now.

In 1972, Deep Purple released an epic song. A song that moved me to sing at decibel levels that resulted in door pounding by my mom, along with "Keep it down. For God's sake. That sounds AWFUL!"

It wasn't just the volume she objected to; it was also my voice. And maybe the words. I dunno. My usual response was to turn the volume dial on the record player—to the right.

Whoa, Cuuuz-innnn Waaah-terrr . . .

And fire in the sky

I heard the song again recently on a Peloton playlist, but this time when I tried to sing along, I couldn't get the words out for laughing. For more years than I'll admit, I honestly thought those were the lyrics. They made sense to me because I've always been very close to my cousins. I thought a cousin named Water sounded earthy and cool, failing to realize the song's title was actually "Smoke on the Water."

Funny thing is, whatever you believe to be true is true. It's *your* truth. Your perception becomes your reality. How do you currently perceive your heart and its voice? Your heart voice is the one that speaks from your soul. It's the voice you were born with. It's pure, and when you listen with your body, you can sense this truth. It's a knowing feeling that's hard to explain scientifically.

Whatever you believe to be true is true.
It's *your* truth.

Heart voice power is what we look for in times of despair, when we don't know what to do, or when something important to us starts to get hard. It can renew our resolve and provide us with lasting sustenance when we're exhausted and overwhelmed. It's what gave me the strength to leave Victimtown . . . after a stay of, ohhhh . . . I dunno, 19,082 days!

Yet, even when we believe in its existence, we still struggle to explain it. Some of the most exquisite things in nature and life are hard to explain scientifically. That doesn't mean they're not there. Beliefs change all the time. I believe in heart voices—yours and mine. Here's my plan.

The Heart Voice Power Plan

1. Put the town voices in their place.

2. Entice your heart voice to get loud.

3. Listen and act on your heart voice wisdom.

It may seem simple, but this three-part plan is a total game-changer. Once you can hear and trust your own heart voice, I want you to turn up the volume and follow its wisdom. You won't be disappointed.

I promise.

CHAPTER 18

Put the Town Voices in Their Place

Nobody can make you feel inferior
without your consent.
—Eleanor Roosevelt

I get it. The voices in our head can be confusing. It's not always easy to sort out which voice is putting a thought into our heads, because the town voices are very tricky. They can sometimes disguise themselves as a heart voice, like the wolf in sheep's clothing. This can cause us to wonder at times, "Is it my heart voice wanting to protect me from criticism? Or is it a town voice trying to hold me back?"

One way to determine which voice is in your head is to consider how it makes you feel. If the thought makes you feel good, that's probably your heart. If it makes you feel anxious or afraid, then for sure it's a town voice. All voices have a motivation. The motivation is either fear or love. Fear includes feelings like frustration, anger, resentment, and shame, or sometimes it can make you defensive. Love includes the fun, happy, relieved, calm, hopeful, and proud feelings.

You can check in with your body as well. The town voices might tell you that something "feels good," and you might actually feel that good emotion in your head when you believe them. But the body doesn't lie. You might not hear the words of your heart voice, but you can always *feel* its response in your body. It won't feel right. You might get a head-ache, upset stomach, or just feel *off* without knowing why. Messages from the town can be felt physically. That's what stress is. When some-thing doesn't feel right in your body, it's a sign that your heart's trying to tell you something.

> You might not hear the words of your heart voice,
> but you can always *feel* its response in your body.

Our heart will always disagree with the town voices. The Boss and her cohorts are shit disturbers through and through. Yep. These voices need a very big smarten-up talk. If you're wondering, "How, exactly, do I have the smarten-up talk with a town voice?" Well, I've got a few ideas, but it's important not to judge yourself, or anyone else for that matter, about how you choose to go about it. Follow whatever strategies, con-cepts, or tips feel right for you in the moment. Although there's no way to get rid of the town voices entirely, we can learn to manage them. The way we put our town voices in their place will be different for all of us.

Fear Is a Pretty Shitty Friend

The majority of us are very rarely, if ever, subjected to life-threatening circumstances. Still, we've likely experienced paralyzing fear at some point in our lives. It's awful. Fear is the main culprit that stops us from taking action—*any* action. It has the power to stop us in our tracks. Fear's also what causes us to take the *wrong* action. When we're scared, we often make choices solely to avoid an unwanted possible outcome.

Other than alerting us to situations where our life is at risk, fear doesn't serve us at all. Think of the regrets you have about your life. We all have at least one. When we acknowledge that our inability to act or talk was due to fear, regret is imminent. The regrets that I have are not about the things that I tried and failed. I don't even regret the times something totally blew up. I regret the things that I didn't do. I regret not taking a chance, not saying what I really meant, not doing what was best for me, not being who I really was. We don't ask someone for a date, because we're afraid they'll say no. We don't speak our truth, because we want to avoid judgment and rejection. These regrets spawn the wonderings of "what if . . . ," and that's a very deep and dark hole, my friends. If you're wondering why you didn't do any of the things that you now regret, the answer is simple: fear.

When relied on as a motivator, our fear can sometimes push us in a direction that's not in our best interest. Fear forces us to think about the short term, about lack, and about worst-case scenarios. Fear is a shitty friend toward our heart and the best friend of the town voices. Fear causes us to do things for the wrong reasons. We enter careers that we don't enjoy because we're afraid that we won't earn enough money doing what we love. We stay in unhealthy relationships because we're afraid to be alone or that we won't have enough money. When we listen to the town voices spew messages of fear, we choose what's (seemingly) safe over our heart's desires. If we let it, fear will hold us back from being who we truly are.

Fear originates in the unknown. When something happens for the first time, or in a new or different way, our brains have no previous information about how to handle it. Without a previous experience to provide a proven meaning, our brain must sort out what this event means. And we now know that our brains don't like a gap in knowledge. Fear is quick to the draw. A voice in our head will readily offer an explanation, as fear loves to tell us exactly what things mean. And the next thing ya know, fear offers us advice and tells us what we need to do to protect ourselves. Fear is our friend when we need to run for our lives, but that's about it.

Knowing all this about fear makes it easier to put the town voices in their place because, without exception, everything they have to say is calculated and designed to make us afraid.

Agree to Disagree

Silencing a town voice completely is not always possible. When this happens, we can agree to disagree. Let the voice say its piece and acknowledge that it's entitled to its opinion. Because, in your heart, you know better. There's no sense ramping up a fight with a town voice that's loud and relentless because that's exactly what it wants. Sometimes, it's easier to surrender to its existence, but with some strict boundaries. The Boss or whichever town voice is talkative is welcome to say what they want. We can choose not to argue. We can decide that it's just not worth pushing back. We might say, "Yeah, okay. I hear you. You can think what you want. I know differently." Personally, I've found this most effective when I talk back to it out loud.

Know Their Motives

The town voices seek to enslave us. Their mission is to uphold and reinforce the three shitty beliefs: I am unlovable, my needs are not important, and the world is unsafe. Victimtown is where they want us to stay; it's where they're in charge. They order us into battle constantly by starting arguments with our heart. Their main strategy is to instill fear in us. Their main mission is to control us. They keep us afraid because that's their only strategic advantage. Listening to them and acting on their advice and directives without questioning their motives is exactly what they want.

I should let you in on something else about these town voices. They don't like to lose, especially if they've been in charge of us for a long time. To that end, they might try to convince us that the last thing we want to do is feel our feelings, especially the hard ones like rejection, loss, and pain. But they don't stop there. They get us to shy away from the good feelings too. They're dirty fighters. They lie. They tell us they're protecting us from hurt. Their advice for us—to avoid intimacy, not take a chance, stifle our voice, or drink away our problems—is only for their benefit, not ours.

Becoming aware of their motives enables us to anticipate their next move. When we question them, they'll invent all kinds of ridiculous rationalizations to keep us afraid. The town voices love linear thinking. They trick us into believing that a certain thing always leads to a certain outcome. It's a catchy attention-grabbing tool they use to trap us. Don't fall for it.

If we're wavering, even a little bit, in our belief about anything, they're ready to pounce. Just when we think we understand how the town voice works, they change tactics. Town voices know how to sideswipe us. They're also capable of completely changing their appearance. They don't always say nasty things. Sometimes, in their most manipulative moments, they play the *good cop game* to trip us up. It can sometimes seem they know us better than we know ourselves. The town voices, however, are just bullies. At their core, they are insecure and in pain. It helps to understand how they operate, and we can take stock in the fact that they are no match for our heart voice. Not even close.

"What If . . ."

The Victimtown voices are masters of "what if . . ." questions. They concoct the most disastrous possible outcomes with an eerie ability to know precisely what will frighten us the most. Regardless of how outlandish or unlikely the scenarios are, if we've been living in Victimtown for a while, we're used to believing them. What-ifs can drive us crazy, because there's no end to the possibilities when we allow a town voice to go on a rant. This is how we can end up in a downward spiral. If we give them an inch, they'll take a mile. Go ahead, you can say it, "The town voices are assholes!"

Here are some of the things I've heard them say: "What if everyone laughs at you?" "What if you get your heart broken again?" "What if people think you're stupid?" "What if you fail miserably, lose all your money and assets, everyone you love abandons you, and you end up living in a cardboard box under a bridge eating cat food?"

The truth is, it's almost never the things that turn out differently than we expect, or completely blow up, that we regret in life. Almost always it's the things we didn't try that we regret. We wonder forever how our life might've been different. That's the ultimate and sad what-if. The what-if of NOT doing or trying or saying something is the hardest what-if to live with. It's so much easier on our hearts to pick up the pieces of a less-than-desirable outcome and keep going than the alternative.

But WHAT IF the town voices are testing us? What if they're checking to see if we've got what it takes to stand up to them? These are valid questions. Those town voices egg us on, like bullies do. When we realize what they're doing, it can make us just mad enough to put them in their place. We can respond with our heart voice and tell them, "Oh no you don't. I know exactly what you're doing." And keep moving forward. We can choose instead to listen to our heart voice 'cause it's got some what-ifs of its own, things like, "What if you really like it and it brings you immense joy?" "What if they think your idea is brilliant?" "What if this brings you success beyond your wildest dreams?"

Voice Your Fears

Most of us think we're the only ones with insecurities and fears. Or that our fears and insecurities are somehow worse, weirder, or more prevalent than anyone else's. Of course, the town voices want us to believe that, but it's just not true. They also tell us that nobody could ever understand our insecurities, which is just another strategy to keep us in Victimtown. Having fears and insecurities is what makes us human. We all have them; the only difference is what they're about and where they lie on a spectrum from mild to severe.

The power that a fear holds over us is lessened instantly by the very act of talking about it. And when we're less afraid, the town voices have much less to say.

Also, when we admit our fears, we'll likely learn that we're not alone. I guarantee you other people exist who share even our weirdest fears, so they can empathize. Comfort and courage can be found in comradery if there's a common goal to leave Victimtown together.

HALT

Each of the town voices has an uncanny ability to pinpoint the most opportune time to start yattering at us. They can sense when we're most vulnerable. But we can be aware, too. An acronym used in recovery, called HALT, is a helpful tool. HALT stands for Hungry, Angry, Lonely, Tired, and it's an easy way for us to identify when we're most susceptible to messages from the town voices.

You can keep one step ahead when you're aware of your weakened state. Their strategic advantage can be eliminated when you take the time to eat, breathe deeply, call a friend, or have a nap. If the voices in your head get out of control, check in to see if any of these states apply. Chances are, if you deal with the aspect of HALT that's relevant, the voices will settle down.

Interrupt Them

Manners are irrelevant and unnecessary when it comes to conversations with the town voices. Don't think twice about just shutting them down.

When a thought pops in your head that makes you feel terrible, you can say, "Shut up," "I'm not listening to you," or "Just stop. I don't want to hear it." When you interrupt it right away, you put that voice in its place before it has the chance to finish its diatribe. It's not rude. Besides, if your town voices are anything like mine, they interrupt us. All. The. Time.

Here and Now

A lot of what the town voices have to say relates to things that haven't even happened yet. When we take a step back and bring in a bit of logic, we'll see that whatever they're saying is NOT actually happening right here, right now. It's also very possible that it may never happen. But even if it does, we'll figure out how to deal with it. It makes no sense to stress about something that hasn't happened. Our heart voice will confirm that *right here, right now, everything is okay.*

Another strategy they use is to tell us our worry demonstrates how much we care. The Monster says that the extent to which we worry corresponds directly with the importance of the issue. The Boss advises us that not only is it our job to worry, particularly about the people we love, but also if we don't worry, it means we don't love them. What a crock of shit! And when we're exhausted from worrying, the Dirtbag will hand us a bottle of wine and tell us we deserve to enjoy a weekend-long, peaceful hike. With Netflix. We've earned it!

How many times have we worried and worried and been so upset about something that, in the end, never happened? We miss out on a lot of life when we're worried and afraid. After the moment has passed, we look back and say, "Wow, that was a colossal waste of time. All that worrying for nothing." Your heart knows this is almost always the case. All that angst can be avoided when we put the town voices in their place right away.

The town voices win battles easily if we choose not to engage. The stakes are high. The stakes are peace, love, freedom, and joy. If we don't learn how to fight this war effectively, we won't stand a chance. It's hard at first. You'll flounder and slip up, as we all do when we're learning something new, but your heart voice will grow as new habits are formed. It takes practice and patience to build up our heart voice power and win battles consistently. The town voices are manipulative, ever evolving, and relentless. This is a war we must be willing to take on for the rest of our lives. Our heart voice is the only one qualified to be the Boss of us.

Our heart voice is the only one
qualified to be the Boss of us.

CHAPTER 19

Entice Your Heart Voice to Get Loud

> You created this moment from what you
> thought and felt three days ago. What you are
> thinking and feeling right now will create your
> next moments. You cool with that?
>
> —Joe Vitale

After we put our town voices in their place, there'll be more space in our minds. This alone gives our heart voice breathing room to play. There are many things we can do to entice our heart voice to speak louder and more often.

Observations from our heart will remind us that we are whole. Our heart voice will confirm we are exquisite in our every human aspect. It will support being nonjudgmental of ourselves and others. When our heart voice gets loud, we begin to believe we're lovable and worthy of our unique place in the world, that our needs are important, and the world isn't meant to be feared.

It's time we realized that our heart voice is here, first and foremost, for us. It wants to be recognized and valued. Our hearts are bursting to share the gifts within that are meant especially for us. Let's give it the positive reinforcement it desires and deserves. The best news is that when our heart voice gets louder, we'll have extra power to share with others.

The Same Way We Help Our Friends

Often, we're kinder to our friends than we are to ourselves. Without hesitation, we offer our friends compassion, understanding, encouragement, support, and acceptance of their mistakes. We respond to their problems with love. When they share the shitty messages in their heads with us, we reply with kind words from our heart. We tell them they're worthy, they're good enough, they deserve the best. Yet, so often we fail to treat ourselves with the same courtesy. The next time a town voice starts talking shit in your head, ask yourself, "If my best friend were saying this out loud to me, what would I tell them?" And then tell that same thing to yourself.

Give It a Formal Invitation

Our hearts can hear us. They hear our every word, both the words we speak aloud and the voices in our heads. And through energetic vibration, our hearts feel the meaning of our words. Our hearts are always listening. They don't miss a thing. If our heart voice has been tamped down for a long time, we may need to give it permission to speak. A formal invitation always gets attention. You can say, "I'm ready to listen to my heart" or "Come on, heart voice. Time to speak up. I want to know what you think." A little reassurance is always well received.

When we're in the middle of a shitstorm, we can ask for its help in whatever way feels natural. I suppose this could be construed as a type of praying, and perhaps it is. Subscribing to any formal religion, however, isn't required to call upon our heart voice. All we have to do is ask. Giving it permission or an invitation may be all it needs for you to hear it. This invitation can be as grand or simple as you desire.

Affirmations

Everyone likes to hear compliments and words of encouragement. Affirmations are one way to compliment, support, and encourage our hearts. Because our entire bodies listen to the voices in our head, affirmations send positive and healing vibes to all of our cells. To make this practice more powerful, we can visualize our hearts, or any body part, healing or growing stronger as we write or recite the affirmation.

For many months I wrote this affirmation out by hand, and I said it out loud every day:

My Daily Affirmation

"There is no one in the world like me.
I am more than enough—exactly the way I am.
My life matters. I am an anti-victim.
I release any remnants of my victim armor daily, and I
stand tall, straight, and light with my heart strong and
wide open.
My heart voice knows best, and I trust it implicitly."

There is an abundance of affirmations online. You can search for particular topics or write your own. Whatever feels like the right fit for you is what it's all about. When used regularly, you'll likely find that you outgrow specific affirmations because your heart doesn't need encouragement for that particular thing anymore. Then you can edit or replace the message for even greater growth.

Feel Our Feelings

The reason we have them, the *purpose* of our feelings, is to provide all the unique and accurate information required to guide us toward our best life. Like a Happiness GPS, remember? Each of our feelings communicates an enlightened intelligence meant specifically for us. Our feelings are messages from our heart that are meant to steer us away from what's not in our best interest and to guide us toward what is. Sometimes the messages are loud and clear. Sometimes our feelings are clues that require further investigation.

Here's the kicker: When we don't acknowledge or take the time to feel our feelings, we miss the message. Missing messages from our heart is what causes us to lose our way. The town voices know how all this works; they don't want us to hear the messages from our heart, so they steer us away from feeling our feelings. We can, however, decide to override them and feel all our feelings any old time we feel like it! And for no other reason than we just feel like it.

Missing messages from our heart is
what causes us to lose our way.

Learning to understand and trust the messages our feelings carry enables us to regulate ourselves and successfully navigate the world. This takes practice and dedication. And courage. It's always fear that holds us back. When we're too afraid to feel, we don't hear the best advice in the whole wide world: the wisdom that comes from our heart. Taking time to really *feel* the feeling, is a requirement for the message to be heard. At times, this can be a very tough ask.

As adults, we might think that we've dealt with our painful feelings over the years. We might genuinely believe that we've released them. Most therapists and psychologists would agree that if we're suffering in any way as an adult, there are likely some hard feelings still festering in our subconscious minds. If they've been left unprocessed for a long time, they've also seeped into our bodies. The Dirtbags will tell us the entire issue is safely locked up in storage and can't affect us while it's there. But they're wrong. Feelings are the leaky, messy part of all issues. Regardless of where we store our shit, the feeling parts of it are held in our very cells. They stay there until we feel them. We must feel the feeling in its entirety and with all of its intensity. Only then can we let it go and be healthy. Feelings are meant to flow through us. They don't want to be stuck inside of us any more than we want them to be. Each and every feeling wants to deliver its message and then keep on going.

The fastest way to release a feeling is to not fight it.

We don't get to choose our feelings. Our feelings choose us, and we must deal with whatever feelings come our way. Many of us, however, try to control our feelings. That's the Boss advising us again. Feelings need to flow naturally on their own schedule and of their own accord. Our contribution is to let them. The path of least resistance is acceptance. We must give up control so they can do what they're meant to do. The fastest way to release a feeling is to not fight it. Engaging in a battle with our feelings is fruitless. "But I don't want to feel sad," never makes us feel less sad. "I don't deserve to be this happy," only erodes our feeling of happiness. We need to fight the town voices, and we also need to succumb to the feelings.

The way we let our feelings perform is by surrendering to them. We let the feeling take over. We decide that it's okay to be sad. We cry for as long as we need to. Once we fully experience the feeling, it will leave on its own. It's impossible to make a feeling leave before it's ready. We can't force a feeling to do anything. There's no telling anyone how long or what it will look like to fully experience a feeling. You must be willing to go along for the ride and trust your heart voice to support you as you go.

One thing we can do when we're on this "feeling" ride is to get curious about the messages. Understanding the meaning will help the feeling dissipate. When we figure out what's behind the anger, it's easier to release it in a healthy way.

Our hearts grow stronger from the workout of feelings being felt and released. Feeling our feelings is the fitness program to keep our hearts healthy. The act of feeling and releasing is the exercise required for our heart to build strength. Healthy, strong hearts have more confidence to speak up. Feelings get validated only when they are felt. This is true regardless of what the feeling is. Validated feelings increase our heart voice power more than anything else. Our heart voice power supports our self-worth. The act of feeling is how we show our heart, with our actions, that we value its advice.

To feel our feelings is the single most important thing we can do. It's the one thing that will shut down the town voices almost immediately. You see, it's our repressed and denied feelings that provide *their* power. Every time we avoid a feeling or slough it off too soon, we strengthen the voices in Victimtown. When we choose instead to welcome our feelings and give them the space and time required, the town voices have no option but to retreat.

I know it sounds hard. It is hard. But it gets easier.

The Shitty Feelings

Emotional pain sucks. Feeling sad is terrible. There's no way around it. Heartbreak is the hardest thing that humans must endure. Loss and rejection can be debilitating. It may take years to overcome tragedy or trauma. Nobody enjoys feeling ashamed or lonely either.

We must tolerate the most intolerable feelings; we must find the courage and strength to sit with them, to give them the validation they deserve, to decode their messages. Only then will the feeling be free to leave us and move on. I'm not saying we should sit forever in our fear and pain, because that's not the answer either. Instead, I invite you to give due attention to these hard feelings, to stop fighting or denying them, to accept and welcome them, and feel them. Your heart will know when it's time to let the feeling go.

Many of us picked up our tendency to deny feelings by watching other people. We saw how hard it was; we witnessed their visible discomfort. We made up a story and told ourselves that we would be well served to find ways to avoid pain. We were wrong, but nobody told us.

Negative feelings have much to teach us about boundaries. We can learn to make connections between circumstances or actions and the feelings we have in response. These connections point out what's best for us. Not what's best for other people—only what's best for us. This knowledge is the foundation of developing boundaries.

Here's the thing: All we can do is the best we can in the moment with the resources we have available. Our best gets better as our most valuable resource, our heart voice power, increases. Feeling our feelings increases our heart voice power more than anything else.

As yucky and heart-wrenching as negative feelings are, they do serve us well. We need them to find our way. They're as much a component of our Happiness GPS as the good feelings.

Feeling our feelings gives us
more heart voice power.

The Great Feelings

It's wonderful to experience emotional highs! We all want to be happy and feel good. Sustained states of awesome feelings reflect the achievement of our yearnings. In the context of our Happiness GPS, feeling great proves that we're on the right path. Our heart is at the helm of our guidance system. It's our birthright to enjoy all the good feelings. Everyone deserves to be happy. And happiness *is* possible for every single one of us. You may still be doubtful. And that's okay. For a long time, I didn't believe happiness was possible either. But it is. You'll see.

The coping mechanism of denying feelings usually doesn't discriminate between the good ones and the bad. Even though we want to experience the positive and wonderful feelings, many of us tend to diminish the good ones too. Sounds kinda stupid, but it happens more than you think. We do this by not embracing every element of the good feeling. We dismiss the bliss by being only a *little bit* excited or proud, and in so doing, we get only a *little bit* of the important message. We get only a *little bit* of all the benefits that go along with reveling in the good feelings.

We're not alone in our inclinations to tamp down the best-feeling feelings. Familial or cultural influences may have led us to believe that delighting in our joy is not appropriate. We may think that we don't deserve the good feeling, and, in our shame, we push it away. We might be embarrassed to feel so wonderful while someone close to us is having a hard time. Or perhaps we're afraid that it won't last. We're terrified that if we get used to this wonderful feeling, it will surely be taken from us abruptly. In our effort to avoid that pain, we dismiss it. We force it away.

Sometimes, we resign ourselves to the fact that feeling good is not sustainable, so we might as well let it go. Perhaps you've heard or thought the following:

> "Life is supposed to be hard."
>
> "Nobody can feel good all the time!"

Please know: All good feelings want to be felt in their entirety, to be celebrated and reflected upon. Every. Single. Time. That is, if we want more of them. Wonderful feelings become more available to us as our heart voice grows.

> **All good feelings want to be felt in their entirety,**
> **to be celebrated and reflected upon.**

Anger

Anger is one of the scariest feelings, but it's also kind of interesting. Like fear, it almost always invokes a strong physical response. What's unique about anger is that our bodies tend to react with an acceleration that's not the case with most other feelings, except maybe sexual passion.

Anger management is big business. My Amazon book search found over 20,000 titles. I think this is very telling about our culture's level of emotional intelligence. Judges are even sending people to anger management programs in lieu of jail time. Not knowing how to handle this feeling leads many of us to believe that we're just better off holding it all in. At least that way we won't do something we might regret. Please don't fall into that trap. Suppressing anger can shorten your lifespan. In the short term, holding anger in can increase your blood pressure. Over time, suppressed anger can cause strokes, heart problems, and cancer. I'm not endorsing angry outbursts. Finding healthy outlets for our angry feelings is essential.

Some might say that our culture has become *anger-phobic*. Anger is often automatically paired with losing control and causing harm. That connection isn't just unfair; it's also not true. Anger doesn't always lead to losing control or causing harm. Still, almost all displays of anger are typically viewed as a weakness of character. Feeling angry is not what anyone aspires to. And releasing our anger, well, that's not something that most of us know how to do—at least not in a way that makes us proud. We're taught, or we come to believe on our own, that anger is unacceptable. Expressions of anger are generally deemed inappropriate, especially in public. So, it's no surprise that we learn to hold it in.

Anger is, however, a very appropriate feeling. It's a feeling provided to us for a reason, just like all the other ones. All feelings carry messages meant unambiguously for us. Anger's no different. Anger can show us that perhaps we need to consider a different path. Anger can also be an indication that we need to implement or defend a boundary. Or it can signal a need to address something painful. There are other meanings as well. The point is, as a feeling, anger is sending us information. The purpose of feeling our anger is to decode the message. After we have an introspective understanding of the message, we can choose an appropriate action.

The purpose of feeling our anger is to decode the message.

If we allow our physical reactions to take over without decoding the message, that's when anger brings us problems. Anger is an excellent teacher. It also can surprise us and lead us into very interesting introspections. When we're aware of its purpose and the importance of the message, we're less likely to succumb to quick reactions. Not only can this help us avoid any harm done, it also provides an excellent opportunity for new insights.

Pain

Pain is a sensation that yells at us. Sometimes rudely. It grabs our attention like nothing else. And it's hard to ignore, which serves its purpose. The International Association for the Study of Pain defines pain as "an unpleasant sensory and emotional experience."[1] But, is pain really a feeling unto itself? What makes pain complicated is that it can be purely physical, like when we're injured, but it can also be emotional, or both. A lot of feelings can become physically painful when the feeling is severe, particularly anguish. Whether it's a feeling or physical sensation, the purpose of pain is to deliver a message. Pain may tell us that we need to slow down, rest, or otherwise take care of our physical bodies. Sometimes pain is trying to point out that something needs to change, that there's an important learning opportunity in front of us. The longer we dodge feeling the pain and the lesson it's carrying for us, the more the pain will persist and the greater it will become. Trust me, I have firsthand knowledge—and it's vital intel. Our best shot at softening this hard feeling is to envelop it with love and compassion for ourselves.

Our bodies have an intelligence of their own. Every one of our cells has a memory. When pain isn't released because we refuse, or we're not able, to feel and process the feeling, it gets stuck in our bodies, and we risk having it resurface at a later point in our life. Like anger, the longer our pain is repressed, the more damage it can do to our bodies.

The ability to feel our negative feelings and to express them are learned behaviors. Most of us didn't have parents equipped to teach these skills, because they also didn't have parents with the knowledge and know-how. But it's never too late to learn, and we can show others.

One of the greatest gifts we can give our children and the people we love is to sit with them in their discomfort while they feel their pain. Just sit and be with them. That's all that's required. Often, that's all any of us need: a little company, a hand to hold, a physical reminder that we're not alone. Only through trial and error can we learn how to process pain for ourselves. Having company and encouragement makes a world of difference.

The reality is this: Until we fully feel our feelings, they won't go away, because they have nowhere to go. Only by letting them fill our mind and body can our heart begin to soften the painful feelings. Only when our heart has melted the rock-hard balls of grief, anger, sadness, and hurt will the pain begin to dissipate and slowly leave us. If the pain isn't completely processed, it will find a place to hide inside us, and we'll have to cover it up in order to manage it.

Until we fully feel our feelings, they won't go away.

Feelings and Responsibility

Friends, bosses, life partners, children, parents, and coworkers—these are some of the people we interact with daily. They all have their own feelings. Who or what can impact their feelings? The answer is everyone and everything. Who's responsible for their feelings? The answer is them. Only them. Not us. Each one of us is responsible for processing our own feelings. Yes, we're also responsible for our actions and our words. But how someone else internalizes them, how someone else feels about our actions or words, that is absolutely not our responsibility. Period.

Each one of us is responsible for
processing our own feelings.

This might require some reflection and reframing, especially if, as children, anyone said things to us like,

"You make me miserable."

"You make me so mad."

"You're making me nervous."

"I'm so disappointed in you."

If we heard these comments from our parents or teachers, chances are we came to believe that we were responsible for how the other person felt. It's time to unlearn that. It's time to look after ourselves and trust that others will do the same.

Sharing our feelings with the wrong people or too soon in a relationship can bring about consequences that the town voices will be excited to reiterate. Our heart will guide us about when and where it's best for us to tell people how we feel. This will become easier when we practice responses that feel natural, such as, "I'm not really comfortable talking about that just yet." Every time we speak our truth about how we feel, our heart voice is strengthened and we gain confidence—regardless of how well it's received by others. It's also how we find our tribe.

Victimtown has many gifts to offer. Through our struggles there, we learn valuable life lessons and become better humans. It's only detrimental when we're stuck there. It's our responsibility to recognize when we're in any of the Victimtown places. Our denied or unresolved feelings are like an anchor that prevents us from leaving Victimtown. Routes out of Victimtown open up when we feel everything, especially the hardest things.

Release Feelings from Our Bodies

When I was in the thick of divorce angst, during that awful period when my husband and I were still living in the same house and *pretending* for

the kids' sake, when we were not speaking and secretly sleeping in different beds, when I'd just taken a new job because I'd been home for
a few years but now needed an income, when I thought I had my shit
together about what was going down and had a workable plan in place
for our new life, something happened on my drive to work.

There wasn't much traffic. I wasn't in a hurry, anyway. And I wasn't
thinking about anything in particular when it started. I stopped at a
red light. While I waited for it to turn green, my vision started to nar-
row. Every little thing in my peripheral vision got fuzzy, and then it all
vanished. Almost like a hallucination, in mere seconds I felt like I was
looking through a peephole, and the single glowing red light was all I
could see. Nothing else existed.

What the hell is happening?

My heart began to pound. I closed my eyes tight and shook my
squinted face to clear my vision. I shook it hard, but when I opened
my eyes, nothing had changed. Rapid fire beats filled my chest.

Holy shit. I'm having a heart attack!

Time slowed in direct proportion to my narrowed vision until it
came to a halt. There was just this moment—a red world, my pounding chest.

I can't catch my breath. Am I having a stroke?

My brain tried to crank. I needed to process what was happening,
but like a dead battery, the motor just wouldn't turn over. Very loud
and unrelenting honks from other cars jolted me back to the reality of
a new world—one that was no longer red but very bright green!

Oh. God. What do I do now?

A divine type of autopilot took over, and I managed to drive ahead
and pull into the first place available—a gas station. I slid the gear into
park, unbuckled my seat belt, and dialed 911.

"Nine-one-one. What's your emergency?"

"I'm having a brain aneurism," I said.

The paramedics who arrived in what seemed like forever but was actually no time flat, were lovely. They checked me out quickly and thoroughly and said, "You're going to be fine."

"I'm not dying?" I said.

"No."

"What's wrong with me?"

"It's acute anxiety. You had a panic attack."

"No. I don't think so. That can't be it. I've got everything under control."

The young paramedic gently tilted her head, lowered her chin, and looked up at me with wide eyes and pursed lips. Silence ensued.

WTF?

Pain, in all of its forms and intensities, is a big wake-up call. There's nothing that gets our attention faster. It screams at us, "TIME TO MAKE A CHANGE, YOU DING DONG!" If we're paying attention, there are great lessons to be found in our pain. I thought I had everything under control. I thought I was dealing with my feelings. My body told me differently.

We're born with only one body. One vessel to serve us for our entire lifetime on earth. Each is unique with features that benefit us and aspects that challenge us. By design, everyone's body is limited or restricted to some degree in some way. Capable of providing both intense pleasure and unbearable pain, we depend on our bodies for a whole lot. We can't truly comprehend this level of dependency until such time as our bodies break down. It's in the Epiphany Hospital that we really get it through our heads that our bodies are single-use instruments.

It's not just our hearts and minds that listen to the voices speaking in our heads. Our entire bodies hear the words too. All the bits and pieces that make up our physical being are listening. And they're reacting. We learn more about what a person really means by watching their body than by listening only to their words. Likewise, we learn more about how we're handling our own feelings when we check in with our body.

Emotions are absorbed into our systems. The ones that are healthy to hold on to like love and joy are visible to others even when we say nothing at all. There's a softness about us that people can see. Pain, anger, and fear are also noticeable in the physical body. People with these feelings can look hard, mean, or defeated.

There's a physical cost to repressing feelings. And it's not just the hard emotions that we lock up. Some of us are afraid to feel the good ones, too. Our cells are smart, but they're not smart enough to understand that the emotions they're holding are from a past experience. Our bodies think it's happening right now in the present moment. Always. Especially when a town voice provides confirmation. As a result, our cells take action to defend themselves. They send warning messages of pain to get our attention, hoping we'll see what's going on inside of us! Stomachaches, headaches, and fatigue are often a demonstration of our cells attempting to get rid of feelings stuck inside of our bodies. The longer our negative feelings are stuck inside, the more damage they can do.

Dr. Bradley Nelson in his book *The Emotion Code* reveals an energy-based protocol to identify and release trapped emotions. By tapping into our subconscious minds, it's possible to rid ourselves of emotions we suppressed as children, emotions we absorbed in utero, and even trapped emotions we inherited from previous generations.[2] Of course, this doesn't excuse us from feeling our feelings going forward.

All feelings have an uncanny ability to show us what we need to learn. Damn. This news is not always easy or nice, 'cause there's a lot of hard feelings out there. There's also the issue of timing. There's never a convenient time to learn a life lesson. Never. It's understandable, then, why we sometimes choose not to feel our feelings. But that doesn't lessen their critical role in our emotional development or happiness.

All feelings have an uncanny ability to
show us what we need to learn.

Clarity

It's pretty cut-and-dried. Clarity is required to hear our heart voice. Respect for our bodies is required to gain clarity. When our senses are dulled, we can't feel anything fully. When we can't feel our feelings, we have no Happiness GPS. Not only are we without our navigation system, but we also effectively cut off our hearts' exercise regimen when we're unable to process our feelings. Without exercise, our heart voice will weaken. And what's more, numbing substances are the preferred fuel for the town voices. The Boss and her cohorts, they all love that shit. Alcohol is at the top of the list for things that keep us stuck in Victimtown.

When we can't feel our feelings, we have no Happiness GPS.

Not that long ago, smoking wasn't bad for us. Not even for pregnant women. Today, everyone knows that smoking is extremely unhealthy. Perhaps one day soon, we'll all concede that alcohol is a highly addictive poison that's responsible for more than 140,000 deaths every year in the US alone.[3] That's 384 deaths per day. Every day. In addition, alcohol causes 30 percent of all deaths on the road. The evidence is mounting—in increments of 384 humans, all with intrinsic value, every day. It's the most prevalent activity in Victimtown.

The corporations with futures at stake are working hard to put their own spin on the evidence. They hire companies to imitate the town voices and promote their products. Their overreaching messages have conditioned us to believe that alcohol is the answer to stress, the means to relaxation, and the essence of pleasure. Society supports those beliefs. Alcohol is the only drug that we have to justify *not* taking. Nobody asks us why we don't smoke cigarettes or use heroin, but they're quick to question why we don't want a drink. Nobody tries to convince us to smoke or shoot up, but they try hard to put a drink in our hands.

In her book *This Naked Mind,* Annie Grace explains how drinking is no longer a fully conscious choice. We've been bombarded for our entire lives with overt and subliminal messages that alcohol will solve all of our problems. Collectively, we perpetuate and reinforce these beliefs with our expectations and judgments among each other. Lastly, to seal the deal, the substance itself hooks us on a physical level with its highly addictive properties to which nobody is immune. Neither weakness nor willpower factor into it.[4]

Alcohol puts our heart voice to sleep and gives all the power to the town voices. It silences our intuition. It takes control of our emotions. When we consume alcohol, we lose the clarity, motivation, and sense of direction required to leave Victimtown.

> **Alcohol puts our heart voice to sleep and gives all the power to the voices of Victimtown.**

The benefits of living a sober life are becoming well known. An ever-growing emergence of accurate data, resources, and new varieties of support are available today for anyone looking to embrace, or just flirt with, sobriety. Grace's book also uncovers "the mystery of spontaneous sobriety." I highly recommend it.

Ommm

The mention of the word meditation has lots of people responding with things like, "Seriously? I've tried it and I can't. My mind is too busy, and what's the big deal about meditation anyway?" Oprah endorses it along with most mental health practitioners. I'll lead with that. And Jeff Weiner, executive chair of LinkedIn, attributes much of his ability to perform under pressure and to think clearly to his daily practice of meditation.[5]

What if I told you that just eight weeks of short daily meditation could actually *increase* the size of the parts of your brain that deal with learning, memory, and emotional regulation? That's what a 2011 study by the University of Massachusetts Medical School found out. After eight weeks, people also experienced less stress and anxiety, less chronic pain, and more general happiness.[6] Other studies show that regular meditation can reverse biological aging. Wow. Who's not up for that?

If that's not impressive enough to give it a try, here's my take on it: You've got nothing to lose and everything to gain, so, seriously, why the hell not? Somehow, it's become a very intimidating endeavor. But wait. Aren't thoughts of intimidation based in fear? Isn't that just a town voice? I was skeptical at first too.

Emily Fletcher, a leading expert in meditation for high performance, said, "The point of meditation is not to get good at meditation; the point of meditation is to get good at life."[7]

Breathing is all it takes to begin to meditate. Sit quietly and concentrate on your breath. Let your mind go wherever it goes without fighting it. Meditation provides the ultimate environment for our heart voice. Without judgment or expectation, give it a whirl for ten minutes.

As a daily practice, or when shit happens like a fly flying in your mouth, if you focus on your breath for a short meditation, your heart voice will show up to help. You may find that just like more cowbell transformed that song in the *Saturday Night Live* skit, meditation can transform your life.

CHAPTER 20

Listen and Act on Your Heart Voice Wisdom

It is our choices, Harry, that show what we truly are, far more than our abilities.

—*Dumbledore*, Harry Potter and
the Chamber of Secrets, *J.K. Rowling*

Our heart voice is our true north. It will never steer us wrong. If there's anything in this world we can trust implicitly, it's that. Particularly if we're afraid, our heart voice will offer a response that will, without exception, lead to a better outcome than any advice we'll get from Victimtown. At one time or another, we've all been afraid of something: being laughed at, someone taking advantage of us, being wrong, being right, being ridiculed, failing, not being loved, being loved too much, what other people think, succeeding, losing, winning, being noticed, being overlooked, being heard, not being heard, saying the wrong thing, being rejected, being misunderstood, being abandoned, being accepted, being weird, or showing our true personality.

We're all afraid of the same things. If you want to disrupt the Shitty

Life Circle, I invite you to do whatever you're afraid of anyway. Take a chance and grow your heart voice. Do it all.

The Hearty Life Circle

We're not destined to stay on the Shitty Life Circle. There's a better way to live. The Hearty Life Circle is an option available to you every single time shit happens. Leading us along the high road to figure things out with love instead of fear, the path of the Hearty Life Circle totally circumvents Victimtown. This scenario leads to healthy coping mechanisms, which provide even more strength to our growing heart voice power.

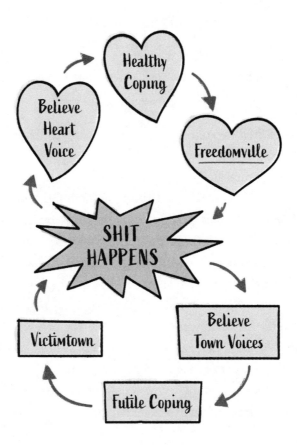

We're either afraid of the experience of doing something or of the outcome. Often, we're afraid of both. We can't stop shit from happening, but we *can* control our response. More than anything else, even more than the severity of whatever shit happened, it's our response that determines the outcome. So, let's look at ways we can be better responders when shit happens.

We're all born with free choice. There are lots of things in life that we can't control, but we always have a choice about how we think. We get to assign whatever meaning we want to any event, comment, or circumstance. The town voices might be loud. Their messages will be crafted to keep us focused on how terrible everything is. But our heart voice is there too. Our heart voice reminds us that our response matters more. Which one will we choose to listen to?

We always have a choice about how we think.

I once got fired by an insecure manager who felt threatened when I uncovered a major error on her part, which caused her to mistakenly think I was after her job. You can bet the town voices had a lot to say about it, too. I was ashamed about the optics, despondent about my future prospects, and terrified of the financial implications. It was bad. As a single mom barely making the mortgage payments, this event caused me tremendous stress and significant hardship, and it confirmed the three shitty beliefs: I'm unlovable, unimportant, and unsafe. I fueled up at the Anger Gas Station, and for many months, I let that manager condemn me to work at the Control Factory, hang out in the Resentment Parking Lot, eat at the Guilt & Shame Café, and spend my leisure time on a worry raft in the Sorrow Swampland.

Today, I look back on this event and see that, although it took considerable time for me to come to terms with it, the firing was the catalyst that launched a new career for me. A career that turned out to be very rewarding. I imagine if I ever run into her, I'll say, "Thank you for being such an insecure bitch. I'm glad you fired me." Then my heart voice would (I hope) make a revision and delete the nasty name-calling part. I can see now that if I'd chosen a different response in the moment, I would've circumvented a lot of the angst. Next time will be different.

One choice we always have in the moment is our own judgment. We can open our minds (and hearts) to the possibility that whatever is happening might not be all bad. It's possible, right? Our hearts understand that every single experience is a chance to learn and grow. It's the Victimtown voices that judge outcomes as bad. Eventually, hindsight will show us what some *shitstorms* really meant. Often, we'll see it was a blessing. But we don't have to wait for hindsight. Our negative judgment in the moment (as advised by one of the town voices) will always get in the way of hearing what our hearts have to say. If, when we're dealing with it, we embrace the possibility of a positive outcome, we won't have to wait for hindsight. Our hearts are full of what I call *nowsight*. Nowsight is what we acquire when we get curious and open ourselves up to the world of possibilities, be they known or unknown. Because the truth is, *anything* is possible.

Nowsight is what we acquire when we get curious and open ourselves up to the world of possibilities, be they known or unknown.

The ability to see events in life without judgment also just makes living easier. Releasing our judgment takes the pressure off. Without the pressure, we're less likely to get all worked up in a negative way or all hyped up in an unrealistic, overly expectant way. Everything that happens doesn't need to be good or bad. It can just be.

The Choice Point

In war, strategic advantages are everything. We must fight the town voices to get out of Victimtown, and we must wrangle with them continuously to stay out. The *pause* is our number-one tactic. The pause holds the *choice point*—the point at which you can either react immediately or take some time to think about it. By capturing, holding, and utilizing the pause, we'll have a crucial strategic advantage.

As a holocaust survivor, Victor Frankl experienced some of the worst things imaginable. In spite of his horrific experience, he returned a very wise and compassionate man, and he's often attributed as having said, "Between stimulus and response lies a space. In that space lie our freedom and power to choose a response. In our response lies our growth and our happiness."

Every time shit happens, there's a point where we get to make a choice. It's the SHIT HAPPENS explosion in the middle of the diagram. I emphasize this only because awareness that this choice point exists is hard to see sometimes, especially when we're in the middle of it. It's not second nature for most of us. Most of us are used to reacting instinctively when shit happens. We've been conditioned to respond without thinking, which is totally normal. Even when we think we've thought about it, we often haven't. Not thoroughly, anyway. A voice in our head is quick to tell us what to do, and until our heart voice is really strong, that voice is typically from Victimtown. The pause is our single, most essential tool. Here's how you can best use it:

> Every time shit happens, there's a point
> where we get to make a choice.

1. **Catch it.** Your first job is to become aware enough to capture the pause. Recognize your opportunity. Thoughtful consideration

(and a lot of practice) is required, as your next steps are going to lead you onto one path or another. Will it be shitty or hearty?

2. **Hold on to the pause.** The town voices will almost instantly bring up your fears. They'll push you to take immediate action. But hold on. Only *you* are in charge of exactly when you're ready to respond. Sure, there might be other people pressuring you or expecting you to do something before you're ready. Tough shit. Make them wait. What's the worst that can happen?? A decision that will land you in Victimtown vs. Freedomville is not a decision to be rushed. Don't let the town voices steal the pause from you. Hold on tight.

3. **Use the pause.** The town voices will tell you that this pause is stupid, unnecessary, or possibly even detrimental to your goals. Hear their messages for what you know them to be and summon your powerful heart voice to defeat them. Then tune in and listen to what your heart says. Believe it. Trust it. Use nowsight and the possibilities it offers as you consider all of your strategic options. Get curious. Reflect calmly on the motivation behind your choices. Discount any options based in fear. Instead, choose a response based in love.

Understanding where your automatic coping mechanisms are trying to lead you and pausing to discern that you don't *have to* go there anymore provides your chance to choose more appropriately. Taking a pause for however long you need, to do anything at all, is your right. Let nobody rush you. Ever. If you get harassed, well, that's what *the hand* is for. For me, the hand means, "Back off and leave me and my pause alone. We'll let ya know when we're good and ready."

The choice is 100 percent yours. You can fuel up in a fury at the Anger Gas Station or mosey over to the Guilt & Shame Café to order up a meal and settle in for the evening. Or. You can pause. You can pause because that's where and when you can hear your heart voice weigh in on the matter. In the pause, you might check in to see if any of the HALT conditions apply (hungry, angry, lonely, tired). Maybe, if you address any of those things, the shitstorm will dissipate.

Healthy Outcomes

I'm a big fan of hiring professionals or asking for help whenever it's necessary. We can't all be good at everything, and it's not the highest and best use of our time to try. This includes therapy. Some issues we can sort out ourselves with the help of books or videos. Other issues, like the ones that need special packaging at the trailhead, may require the help of someone with specific qualifications. And that's okay. I think pretty much everyone could benefit from a therapist at some point in their lives.

The healthy outcomes arrive only when we rely on our heart to gauge our own needs and enlist whatever support or resources will serve us best. It's important to appreciate the value in being gentle with ourselves through this process. We all have numerous problems. It may be more manageable to work on our issues one at a time. With multiple circumstances or behaviors that we'd like to change, our hearts will remind us to be patient and trust that progress and confidence will certainly arrive.

The healthy outcomes arrive only when we rely on our heart to gauge our own needs.

I totally get it. We all want results NOW! Immediate and easy solutions sell for big bucks. However, they rarely work. To take on multiple issues and rip all of our armor off at once requires the appropriate support setting—like what was offered at The Place. Taking off our armor in smaller bits at a time is also a winning strategy. Only you know what the best approach will be. Listen to your heart.

One issue at a time, we can choose to figure things out in new and healthy ways. I wish I could tell you that it'll be easy. The reality is that it's hard, but not forever. The reward for this hard work is the healthy outcome that make us feel good about ourselves. Isn't that the whole purpose of life? Isn't that what we're yearning for? Peace, love, freedom, and joy?

Healthy outcomes aren't always what we expect. Invariably, there are surprises in store for us. Sometimes the healthy outcome is to view other people or circumstances in a different way. Or it may be a new level of understanding about ourselves. Getting clear about what we don't want in our lives also counts as progress. It's just as healthy to sort out what doesn't work for us as it is to discover what works best.

All of these healthy outcomes add up. They serve to strengthen our heart voice. We gain confidence and begin to enjoy a momentum that feeds our expectation of more good things to come.

Surviving a Rogue Wave

We rarely can predict when tragedy might strike like a rogue wave. The Aussies, they know how to do deal with these waves. They've figured it out because rock fishing is a popular, fun sport. They have these life jackets that are flat. They're uninflated and come with CO_2 cartridges that ignite when they get wet. This way, the fisherman's movements aren't inhibited like they would be wearing a traditional life preserver, and the fishermen have a better chance at surviving a rogue wave. Heart voice power provides us with similar protection.

If you want to spend more time in Freedomville, there are things you can do that will help you stay on the Hearty Life Circle. These things include practicing radical self-care, being kind and compassionate toward yourself and others, doing your best, speaking your truth, forgiving others and letting go, and allowing yourself to feel all of your feelings.

If you find yourself slipping onto the Shitty Life Circle, you'll notice you're likely judging more, trying to change or control others, not asking for what you need or want, numbing your pain, or acting impulsively. When this happens, practice the pause and tell those town voices to go take their own hike on the Denial Trails.

In Victimtown, we're powerless. We're searching endlessly to fulfill our yearnings, but we're frail, and if we're stuck there, our efforts are ineffective. We're brainwashed to believe that our power must be obtained. True power, however, cannot be found externally. And it certainly doesn't exist in Victimtown. The power to change, to achieve all that we yearn for already lives inside us. It's the wisdom in our hearts. Heart voice power isn't something we obtain but rather something we grow and release. And, like all other worthy endeavors, there's always some practical shit required to achieve our goals.

Also, please don't feel bad if you find yourself returning to Victimtown from time to time. Visits to Victimtown are unavoidable. It's inevitable that you'll return to heal or learn another lesson. Life's all about balance. The goal is to work toward spending more and more time in Freedomville.

Heart voice power isn't something we obtain, but
rather something we're meant to grow and release.

PART 4

Freedomville

CHAPTER 21

Get Radical About Self-Care

Self-care is giving the world the best of you,
instead of what's left of you.
—Katie Reed

Freedomville isn't freedom from shitstorms. Sorry. I wish it was, but that's not the way it works. Living in Freedomville is all about the freedom to choose how to respond when shitstorms happen and the awareness and knowledge of how and why to make that choice. It takes effort to live here. Some days it takes more effort than others. You'll find a more simple and kind way of living in Freedomville. Competition doesn't exist, and we're no longer yearning, because we like the conversations in our heads. Our lives may not be exactly the way we want, but we trust that we're headed in that direction, that we're on the right path, as we plot the course of our dreams.

First Things First

The first stop in Freedomville is self-care. Self-care is a hotly debated topic. It's often misconstrued. A mainstream perception is that self-care is selfish and that selfishness is a negative quality. Selfish acts are often interpreted as doing things for ourselves *instead of* doing things for others. All of us who grew up believing that our needs weren't important, or at least not as important as the needs of others, well, we usually have a tough time wrapping our heads around self-care.

It's appalling that in many cultures the state of *burnout* has become respected. In Victimtown, it's also revered. It's viewed as something of value. It's a state that's been earned. All the people in Victimtown admire this achievement. Working more, working harder, at the expense of ourselves, is demanded by the Boss and expected by our peers. The Monster loves to create martyrs. Many of us say we're cautious of becoming burned out, but we don't do anything about it, because the town voices reiterate the mandate. When we're not able to keep up, the Maître D' will ridicule us. When we fail to achieve the desired outcome, the Boss will reprimand us. That's because there's no winning in Victimtown.

The Healing Power of Food

Unknowingly, many of us have deprived ourselves for too long. But now that we have a new lens about self-care, it's time to change all that. Let's start with the fundamentals, our basic human needs. One of these is food. We've heard it a million times before, and it's kind of a no-brainer. You are what you eat. Food can heal. Preservatives cause cancer. Blah blah blah. But did you know that diet has a direct impact on our mental health? Are you aware that what we eat plays a role in our feelings of anxiety and depression? Well, it's true. Food affects our feelings and our mood. Our diet affects our ability to cope.

We understand eating well for the benefit of our body. We know about cholesterol and fats as well as the good and bad kind of both. We get the direct correlation between diet and the health of our organs, bones, and muscles. But what about our brain? Our brain is the most complex organ in the body. It would make sense then to take into account the ideal fuel required to keep this baby performing at its best.

A healthy brain enables us to function with higher levels of focus and clarity. A healthy brain is better equipped to respond to life's challenges. It's also not as susceptible to disease. One of my biggest fears is getting dementia. I'm not saying that this terrible affliction can be eliminated with the right diet, but studies do demonstrate irrefutable evidence of the diet–brain connection. Personally, and maybe because I'm a bit paranoid about this possibility, I'm willing to take seriously anything that might help me avoid deteriorating cognitively.

Dr. Eva Selhub confirms that diets high in refined sugars are harmful to the brain. If substances from processed or refined foods get to the brain, the brain has little ability to get rid of them.[1] Multiple studies have found a correlation between a diet high in refined sugars and impaired brain function and even a worsening of symptoms of mood disorders, such as depression.[2]

I get it—radical dietary changes are tough to implement. We don't have to completely overhaul our diet all at once, though. We can start small. Each little choice we make will add up. And it will make a difference.

The Benefits of Sleep

The US Centers for Disease Control and Prevention (CDC) has labeled the problem of adults getting inadequate amounts of sleep a "public health epidemic," and this was before the real epidemic hit.[3] In times of COVID-19 or any other ongoing stress, quality sleep is even more imperative. Sleep is essential for mental and physical health. The number of US adults who sleep less than six hours a day nearly doubled from 38.6 million to 70.1 million between 1985 and 2012.[4]

What's keeping us up? For a lot of us it's the town voices. The Boss, the Maître D', and the Swamp Monster, for example, delight in keeping us up all night. TV, social media, video games, work, phone apps, and one of my personal favorites—NETFLIX binging—are all activities directed by the Dirtbags. Whatever is preventing quality sleep is a problem. Technology and the recent movement to work from home have thrown many of us into an arena where we're expected to be available 24/7. Burnout, here we come!

While it may seem that losing sleep isn't such a big deal, the effects can go way beyond daytime drowsiness. Sleep is essential for our brain health. Deep and regular sleep improves our memory, helps prevent elevated levels of stress hormones, lowers blood pressure, and (as an added bonus) enables easier weight maintenance. Lack of sleep can affect our judgment, coordination, and reaction times. Just think about that for a minute. The implications of reduced capacity for those qualities are huge.

It's during sleep that our brain processes all that's happened in our day. Our brain needs time to recover before we ask it to work again. Every day, we rely on our brains to effectively solve problems, make decisions, negotiate, and perform our work.

Adults need between seven and ten hours of sleep a night. "Not me," you say? Perhaps. There is a small group of people who possess a rare gene that allows them to function well on six hours of sleep a night. However, researchers at the University of California in San Francisco discovered that this gene exists in less than 3 percent of the population.[5] So, for the other 97 percent of us, six hours of sleep doesn't cut it. It's usually a memo from the Boss that says we have this gene, but she's a liar.

Quality sleep does more than restore our brain capacity. Our subconscious minds are ready, willing, and able to work behind the scenes and find solutions, but we need to give them the opportunity. You may be surprised to learn the immense capacity for our hearts to resolve feelings and find solutions for problems while we sleep. Without the distractions of the world, our hearts and brains are able to focus and work together more efficiently. Together, they come up with new pathways, directions, and creative ways to get out of Victimtown.

Give Up the Sauce

There's one single substance that causes more brain damage than almost everything else *combined*. You might not be happy about what that is. But I'm going to tell you anyway.

It's alcohol.

Even in small quantities.

Even if it's only ingested once in a while.

We've been unconsciously conditioned to believe that alcohol will provide friendship and romance, make us cool and courageous, and basically solve all of our problems and make us happy. I call bullshit. Although it's almost impossible to avoid this conditioning, you can absolutely change your beliefs about it.

When we consume alcohol, our brains change. Alcohol does this by interfering with our neurotransmitters and the way our brain functions. It slows down all of our responses. We actually think more slowly. Alcohol deadens our senses and prevents us from feeling. And worst of all, it mutes our heart voice altogether.

I invite you to experience your life without alcohol. No commitment, no judgment—just one day at a time. You think you're smart and articulate now—just wait! After giving up my two to four glasses of wine most nights (okay, definitely more on weekends), I was blown away with the cognitive improvements that were bestowed upon me. And, to my surprise, the brain remodeling continued for about a year! The benefits of giving up the sauce are so much more than just about our brain. In my case, every aspect of my mental health was greatly improved. Once you see the transformative impact of sobriety for yourself, you'll understand.

Get Out

I have a friend that likes to say, "Nature is good dope." And it really is, on so many levels. Think of the comfort, relief, and calm that we enjoy when we're looking at, or when we're in, an element of nature. It's unmistakable. Each of us resonates in a special way with some part of nature. What does it for you? The mountains? The forest? The lake? The beach? The prairies? The desert? The caves? The ocean?

Spending time immersed in nature quiets our mind. The outdoors has a natural way of shutting up those pesky town voices. It's kind of like meditating. When we spend time in nature, the incessant chatter in our heads takes its own deep breath and settles down.

In times of unpredictability and high stress, we all crave comfort and relief. And nature is always there, waiting to restore us. It has a great healing capacity for our physical and mental health. Many studies around the world have shown that recovery times are reduced for patients and that they experience fewer complications if they can see trees from their hospital beds. They actually heal faster. Clearly, on a cellular level, our bodies are replenished by nature's energy.[6]

The term *grounded* is used to describe someone who seems to have their shit together. They have emotional intelligence and appear to have an understanding and acceptance of who they are. Their grounded-ness is an admirable quality. Sheldon Cooper, from the TV series *The Big Bang Theory*, and my best friend Deb, would both agree there are lots of times when a literal interpretation is just the ticket. Getting grounded (also called grounding or earthing) can happen when we put our bare feet onto nature: grass, rock, the forest floor, a sandy beach, the dirt of a field or the meadow—all will suffice. It's about the physical connection. We are one with nature. When our skin touches it, the energy of nature seeps into us. If we close our eyes and imagine the bond between ourselves and whatever we're standing on, it's possible to sense our connection to everything.

Our magnificent planet is free for everyone to savor. It wants to give back to us, too. We need only to be willing to connect. Lastly, when we know how to ground ourselves, we can use it to steady us when we need it most, like the pause of a shitstorm.

Time to Get Radical

Self-care, while a vital part of our overall well-being, is different for all of us. What's important to you? What are the special things that make you feel good? What brings you joy? What do you love doing? Your feelings provide clues. Laughter, satisfaction, gratitude, love, joy, and a feeling of belonging—all these and more can show you what you need to do to look after yourself. Whatever works for you, make a plan to keep yourself filled up, because radical self-care replenishes your resources. It makes you more resilient and able to cope if a shitstorm is sucking the energy out of you.

We've all got a million items on our to-do lists, but we've also got the power, and the responsibility, to prioritize. Radical and regular self-care enables us to trust ourselves. When we can count on ourselves to stay strong and attend to our needs, not only do we like ourselves more, we also implicitly trust in our abilities to handle life when it gets hard. We begin to believe that we've got what it takes, so we worry less. And lastly, on a cellular level, radical self-care is how we tell our heart that we value it, by giving a consistent boost to our heart voice power.

If you're not yet inclined to practice radical self-care for your own sake, there's another way to look at it. What if self-care enabled you to give more to others? What if looking after yourself first was actually in service to others? Most of us have people in our lives that we want or are required to help. To do this we need the bandwidth to listen, be empathetic, patient, or even just available in whatever way might be necessary. Looking after others is a wonderful and generous endeavor, but not when it's at the expense of ourselves. Some of us have no choice in caring for others; parenthood is one example. Self-care isn't just an option. Self-care is a requirement if we want to ensure that we have the resources available to care for others.

By practicing radical self-care, we stay rich with love and compassion, and that's a gift to the world. The more we love ourselves, the more love we have in our emotional bank accounts to share and give to others. Sounds like a win-win to me.

By practicing radical self-care, we stay rich with
love and compassion, and that's a gift to the world.

CHAPTER 22

Forgiveness Feeds Our Yearnings

There is no one greater or lesser than you.
There are only those who have learned how to
reveal their gifts to a greater or lesser degree.
—*James Van Praagh*

For years I hated my ex-husband—nineteen to be exact. While I was working on forgiving him, I came across a Wikipedia entry that stated, "Forgiveness is the intentional and voluntary process by which one who may initially feel victimized undergoes a change in feelings and attitude regarding a given offense and overcomes negative emotions such as resentment and vengeance."[1]

That sounds about right. And that's exactly what I tried to do many times over those nineteen years: books, therapy, and all the new-fad forgiveness exercises—I did them all. But not much changed until three days before I left The Place, when I was asked a question by my therapist in a group session. It was a seemingly random question, directed at me and perfectly timed to arrive only after many weeks of intensive therapy where I'd finally worked through all the shitty feelings that I'd repressed about my marriage. A question that, had it been asked sooner, would've resulted in *the hand*, followed by an irrevocable door slam that any decent card-carrying INFJ (Introverted, Intuitive, Feeling, and Judging personality) is capable of.

She asked me point blank, "What happened in *his* childhood?" Group silence ensued. It wasn't the awkward, eye-contact-avoiding kind of silence that you might expect. Instead, our collective silence had evolved into a supportive, eye-contact-making silence that was introspective for all of us. It exemplified our comfort level with each other and, more importantly, with the therapeutic *bombs* that were regularly dropped in each of our laps.

As that poignant question hung out there, awaiting my response, turmoil was raging in my head. And also, *Why don't they serve wine here? Therapy would be so much better with wine.*

Five minutes went by. I was determined, resolute in my position: *I don't want to talk about this.*

Another ten minutes ticked away.

It didn't matter. Extended silence stopped being awkward weeks ago. Therapists have patience out the ying-yang! A single tear escaped, and more were threatening as I turned to look at Jace, my comrade in arms, sitting beside me. He'd become like a brother to me. As he silently passed the Kleenex box, his eyes said, "You got this."

And then he spoke, "Is it possible that perhaps—just perhaps—he was so conflicted and confused by his own unprocessed pain that he acted the way he did?"

In that moment I wondered what shitty beliefs he adopted. What trauma did he endure that produced the coping mechanisms that he still clings to? That was enough for me to put my grudge bullhorn down and let years of resentment go.

Forgiveness is impossible when we're parked in the Resentment

Parking Lot. I don't know everything that happened in his childhood, or the rest of his life for that matter. And I don't need to. Accepting possibilities (known and unknown) was enough to let me drive out of the Resentment Parking Lot that day.

A Forgiveness Formula

While it's easy to believe in theories—especially honorable ones like intrinsic human value—it's never as easy to apply them to our own circumstances and lives. Walking our talk is the ultimate test. In the situation regarding my ex-husband, I realized if *my* childhood was not *my* fault, then it's only fair that the possibility exists that *his* childhood was also not *his* fault. When I considered the possibility of his pain and his own repressed stuff, something surprising occurred. A feeling I hadn't had toward him in a long, long time surfaced: compassion. Then I wondered about another possibility. If I completely forgave him, what positive implications might that have for our children? I didn't know it then, but it was surely my heart voice that helped me consider things from this perspective. I created this formula to help others and also to remind myself. I call it C-squared (C^2).

C^2: A FORGIVENESS FORMULA

CURIOSITY x COMPASSION = FORGIVENESS

It's pretty straightforward. Curiosity when combined with compassion equals forgiveness.

How can it not?

I hear you. Some things are harder to forgive than others. And everyone is only ready to do this work when they're ready. We can be ready sooner when we get curious and ask questions. Then ask more questions. The answers will likely surprise you and lead you toward compassion.

Forgiveness Is Not Forgetting

Forgiving someone doesn't mean that we have to forget the painful event. Some experiences leave permanent scars on our hearts. These scars are our badges of life. They make us who we are. We all have some. When scars remain, they can remind us of what we've overcome and of what we've learned (albeit, the hard way). It's the process of forgiveness, however, that heals our open wounds.

After we've forgiven, the memory of the painful event adopts a different energy. Yes, it happened. Yes, it was hurtful. But when it's been infused with curiosity and compassion, it changes. When you think about something AF (this time I mean After Forgiveness, not what you thought), it doesn't carry the same weight. It's lighter. It no longer evokes the stinging emotions and pain that it did before. The open wound on our heart is now closed, allowing us to carry on with a new-found strength that makes the memory manageable. We can do this for ourselves without excusing the perpetrator. All forgiveness is ultimately for our own benefit, which is why it's crucial that we also apply the C^2 forgiveness formula to ourselves.

Forgiving Ourselves

It might take a variety of tactics to get curious about ourselves. An objective lens could be activated by asking people we trust. Evaluating measurable results can be helpful, too, if that applies. It often requires a little more effort to be compassionate with ourselves, but that's where our heart voice power comes in. You know all about that now.

Forgiving ourselves is the essence of self-help. The reality is we can't change what's already happened. All we can do when we totally F-up is to do everything in our power to make things right, learn from our experience, and forgive ourselves. We'll be stuck in Victimtown until then. Not one single person on the town council wants us to forgive ourselves because when we do, their power will be diminished. Not only will we no longer be susceptible to their shitty messages about that issue, but also new paths to Freedomville will instantly appear.

It's time to forgive yourself.

For everything.

> It's crucial that we also apply
> the C^2 forgiveness formula to ourselves.

Mistakes and Failures

A significant mistake or failure can swiftly land us in Victimtown. Pick a place, any place! It's a Victimtown law that all mistakes and failures are bad. And punishable. If we had any childhood trauma around making a mistake, this belief is even more ingrained.

Covering up our mistakes or failures is a common coping mechanism from childhood. Okay sure, we might share a distorted story for a little laugh, but guess where that happens? The Denial Trails. Grudges and resentments aren't held only against others; we hold them against ourselves, too. If we let her, the Boss can task us with a never-ending and impossible project she says is designed for us to overcome our failure. If we completely hide our mistakes, especially from ourselves, they fester like repressed emotions and provide essential nutrients for the Swamp Monster. If we end up in the café, the Maître D' turns our failures and mistakes into vomit and serves them to us on a plate. Pretty gross, right?

Get Curious

Forgiving ourselves for actions taken out of anger can be challenging, but curiosity is useful both in the moment and afterwards. When we have the awareness to stop for a minute and explore why we're feeling so angry, we're onto something. By removing self-judgment about our anger, we can observe the experience with detached interest and playful curiosity.

When you find you're having trouble forgiving yourself, get curious and try to figure out what the problem is. For example, ask yourself what triggered this angry emotional response? Has a boundary been crossed? If so, explore what it is about that boundary and its importance to you. This intel might help you establish a new boundary or learn a better way to defend that one.

Anger's an emotion that takes a lot of vulnerability to address. Curiosity changes the focus and gives us a chance to calm down. The things that make us the angriest are usually very personal or shameful. What if we approached anger more gently, like an old friend? "Hey. Haven't seen you in a while. What's going on?" When we welcome an emotion, especially a hard one like anger, we can take care of it. With curiosity, we can show it love and soothe it like we would a crying baby.

Another reason to become curious is that curiosity sparks our imagination, and our sense of what's possible expands. Curiosity takes contemplation. It also requires brainstorming—both of which have a calming effect. Wondering why certain things keep happening or not happening is a way we can start the curious thinking. When you're at a loss for how to be curious, try just saying, "Well . . . isn't this interesting . . ." and see what comes up.

When we don't want to think about something, let alone talk about it, that usually indicates it's exactly what we need to investigate most. Just sayin'.

> What we don't want to think about is usually what
> we need to investigate most.

Embrace Your Mistakes

Many of us learned at an early age that it's best to avoid mistakes and failures. We might've been ridiculed by our peers or punished by our parents. Even worse, children who were punished *and* ridiculed by a parent learned that anyone who makes a mistake or falls short of the mark is a fundamentally flawed person.

We can't grow or learn if we don't make mistakes. Without mistakes and failures, we are stagnant. But there's a catch: Mistakes are valuable only when we acknowledge them. The truth is mistakes are awesome! People who embrace mistakes are brilliant! Mistakes expose all kinds of insights and constructive information for our benefit. Almost never do we get anything right the first time. Everyone who's achieved greatness did it by embracing the mistakes they made along the way. If we choose to view our mistakes as essential and unavoidable learning tools, we'll get to where we want to go faster. And when we're grateful for having made the mistake, when we appreciate the intel, we'll be propelled far beyond our goals because gratitude powers up our heart voice.

By sharing our mistakes publicly, we offer the gift of inspiration to others, and we pave the way for them to do the same. Courage is contagious, and being open about our mistakes is one way to pay it forward. I think all mistake-makers deserve to be revered, ourselves included. I'm going to suggest we even take it a step further. Let's celebrate our mistakes. Let's revel and laugh and learn as we celebrate every mistake or failure for the progress it really is. Imagine how transformative it would be for children to learn that mistakes deserve to be celebrated. How fast and fun the learning process would become!

The voices of Victimtown judge outcomes as either good or bad, but our hearts know otherwise. It's in the messy middle ground where our growth occurs. We deserve the opportunities that exist only in a space without judgment because that's where the possibilities are endless. Often, the information gleaned from a mistake or failure is our heart voice suggesting a better approach, a higher goal, or even a different path altogether—and that's a good thing!

> **Mistakes and failures fortify our
> intrinsic human value.**

We've all made mistakes. And we've all had failures, big and small. And we're all gonna have more. That's what makes us human and our value intrinsic.

Transforming Our Past

Truth in a court of law is one thing. How we choose to interpret our life is up to us. The stories we tell about ourselves and our experiences depend 100 percent on which voice we believe. When we were kids, we didn't know any better when we were making up meanings. But that's not the case anymore. Now that we know how Victimtown and Freedomville work, it's our responsibility to be intentional about the meanings we apply. When shit happens, we're equipped to make a more informed and perceptive choice about what it means. The town voices are eager to tell us what to think, and they're usually the first to speak up. We can rely instead on our heart to figure it out. It may take a bit longer, but our heart has an opinion too. We get to choose which version we believe. And which one we tell others. And when we're able to hear our heart's version, we can rewrite the stories of our past.

Just because we've thought of something one way for many years doesn't mean we can't change our minds (or our hearts). We can adopt a new meaning about whatever happened. In fact, if the event is still painful for us, we must. Here are some examples:

REWRITING OUR STORIES

VICTIMTOWN VERSION: I was so weak, pathetic, and depressed that I needed in-patient treatment. I'll still have to battle depression every day for the rest of my life.

FREEDOMVILLE VERSION: My mental health took a significant turn for the worse, so I got proactive and found the treatment I needed. It transformed my life. I have new insights and strategies I can use if I feel depressed again.

VICTIMTOWN VERSION: That asshole made me so mad that I smashed the window. I couldn't help it. He's lucky I didn't smash his face.

FREEDOMVILLE VERSION: I'm not proud of how triggered I got and the damage I did. I'm working on better responses.

Whatever stories make up our history, we can decide which perspective serves us best. Do we want a version based in fear or a new version founded in love? That decision determines whether we're hanging out in Victimtown or Freedomville. When we can tell our stories to ourselves or others and not feel ashamed or angry or resentful, we've found the version that's based in love. It's a version that feels good (or at least better) to *own*, and that's how we know it's the right one. Sometimes it takes several iterations to get there. And that's okay. **When we own our stories, they no longer hold any power over us.**

What people think or say can no longer embarrass us or make us feel ashamed. When our previous mistakes and old destructive behaviors no longer define us, well, that's freedom.

Rewriting the stories of our childhoods provides new insights and strength to overcome any coping mechanisms we brought into our adult lives that aren't helping us. We can rewrite the meaning of any-thing that happened and start over any day we want. Oh, and in case you were wondering, we can also redefine anything we want, any day we want, including our boundaries.

When we own our stories, they no longer hold any power over us.

CHAPTER 23

Design Your Life with Boundary Basics

May the force be with you.

—*Obi-Wan Kenobi,* Star Wars *(1977)*

B oundaries define what's acceptable and what's not in our lives. They're how we specify our limits for everything and where we draw the line. Establishing, expressing, and defending our boundaries is how we honor our heart voice wisdom. Our hearts are boundary experts. We've worked hard to increase our heart voice power, but we need to do more than listen if we want to find peace, love, freedom, or joy. We must implement the knowledge our heart voice provides. One way we do this is with boundaries.

> Establishing, expressing, and defending our boundaries is how we honor our heart voice wisdom.

Boundaries benefit ourselves and others. Boundaries are about protecting and sharing our personal resources: our love, our time, our bodies, our environment, our knowledge, our money, and our things. We each have our own boundaries. Our unique boundaries benefit both ourselves (protecting) and others (sharing). The limits we define for anything are personal. They're also subject to change. We change them when our beliefs or values are altered (like when we ditch a shitty childhood belief). We adjust our boundaries to reflect new insights when we evolve (like when we rewrite a story about something that happened). Occasionally, under special circumstances, we loosen them. Although boundaries give us a glimpse into what other people value and believe, their purpose is not to control anyone else.

The Boss will tempt us to judge boundaries, other peoples' or even our own. Boundaries aren't good or bad. They are, however, an accurate reflection of how much heart voice power a person has in that particular moment. They can also be scary AF (this time it *is* what you think). They can be forbidding to establish, awkward and vulnerable to express, and exhausting to defend. But boundaries also empower us. They are instrumental in determining how we'll be treated by others.

Setting Boundaries

What we need to set healthy boundaries are an accurate awareness of who we are and how we feel about our resources. I know, you're saying, "Easier said than done." And you're right, because the town voices hate boundaries. They've got a lot to say, and all of it's intended to make us afraid. The Victimtown voices tell us that we'll have no fun, no love, no success, and no happiness whatsoever if we embrace boundaries. Hogwash. Finding the right balance of protecting and sharing our resources helps keep us in Freedomville.

Healthy boundaries will keep us off the Shitty Life Circle and out of Victimtown when shit happens. Our heart voice is equipped with all the intel necessary to set the boundaries that are right for us.

If you're starting from scratch (like I was), I invite you to begin with something where the stakes aren't too high. Take for example, when to say no. Yes, there are times when saying no can have huge consequences. Start with a scenario where that's not the case. Give some thought as to what factors you need to evaluate to set your boundary, and what's important to you. You can also assess what the person is asking (easy vs. hard for you), the time involved, and your enjoyment of the task. These are just a few of the many possible considerations. Only you can evaluate the factors and your feelings to define the criteria to determine where you'll draw the line. You're allowed to say no whenever you feel like it—and for no other reason than you just feel like saying no. Start small. Your confidence will grow. Saying no is the foundation of all boundaries. It's kind of ironic that it's also frequently the first word uttered by humans. By feeling your feelings as you go, you'll soon be able to work your way up to setting boundaries for all of your valuable resources.

Setting boundaries is something you do by yourself. For yourself. It's not really something other people can provide advice about (except, perhaps your therapist). Trying out different boundaries to see how they feel will help you know yourself on a deeper level. It doesn't matter where you draw the line about your love, your time, your body, your environment, your knowledge, or your resources. What's important is that your boundaries are based in love and not fear. This will be confirmed by your heart voice and also by your body. Healthy boundaries *feel* right.

Healthy boundaries *feel* right.

Expressing Boundaries

People are not mind readers, so we're responsible for expressing our boundaries clearly. Through trial and error, we make progress to learn the best time, place, and words to express a boundary. The variables are as endless as human personalities. It takes practice. And courage. And more practice. These three components are a guideline that I used to become more comfortable with expressing a boundary.

THREE BOUNDARY COMPONENTS

1. Your feeling

2. The requested action

3. The outcome you want

The components can be said in any order, for example:

"I feel _____ when (this happens). Would you please _____?"

"When (this happens), I feel _____. I'd rather you _____."

Ultimately, you can't control how others react. Any negative reactions you get when expressing boundaries could be an opportunity to make improvements for the next time. The outrageous and disastrous outcomes that we fear rarely happen. But if they do, it could mean that the boundary is even more essential for your well-being.

Defending Boundaries

From time to time, people cross our boundaries. This can happen deliberately, unknowingly, or accidentally. We can usually overcome any damage right away by pointing it out if we receive the appropriate concern or an apology. However, a deliberate boundary violation is malicious and must be defended in no uncertain terms.

Our ability to defend a boundary varies. We do the best we can with the resources available to us at that time. Our number one resource is our heart voice power. Other resources include our physical health, the time we have available, our brain power, and emotional bandwidth, along with the support at our disposal (such as money and people).

If we have to defend the same boundary more than once with someone, we might consider adding consequences to our boundary statement such as, "When you yell at me, it makes me afraid and angry. I'd rather you walk away and come back when we can talk civilly. If you can't do that, I will walk out myself." Bear in mind, if we add a consequence, we must be prepared to act on it every single time, or we'll be back to square one.

Defending boundaries can be exhausting, and sometimes it feels like it's sucking the life out of us. And it kind of is, because defending boundaries depletes our heart voice power at an expediential rate. I believe this boundary testing happens to show us what we need to learn or heal. We all have to defend our boundaries; that's just a part of life. But if we have to do it all day, every day, we'll be back in Victimtown before we know it.

It's hard to defend boundaries when we want to be accepted. There could be serious consequences when defending boundaries with people we love. The more the relationship matters to us, the more vulnerable we are. Here's the thing though; when the boundary is founded in your core values, you'll attract like-minded people. And when the boundary is founded in love and feels right for you, the people who truly love you will accept it (or learn to). And if they don't, wouldn't you like to know sooner rather than later? Yes, it's sad to end a relationship or not be included. At the same time, our boundaries help us attract the people with whom we're able to share the deepest connections.

Loving with Detachment

Boundaries are hard enough when it comes to the people we love. When someone we love is struggling and needs our help, everything about our boundaries can be easily blurred by the town voices. If the stakes are high, we need to rely on our heart voice more than ever. Loving with detachment is a way to have boundaries around helping people we love or people we're responsible for. We can set, express, and defend our limits to protect and love ourselves while we continue to love and support others. Loving with detachment allows us to do this without ever abandoning them, even when our limits are reached.

An example is not accepting responsibility for their mistakes or trying to rescue them. This is so, so hard—especially as a parent—but it can also be our greatest gift to them. It's a tough concept to embrace, but loving with detachment is how we increase the heart voice power of our children. It's hard because, in order to do this, we must watch them struggle as they learn. We practice loving with detachment by not fixing or controlling everything in their lives. By not rescuing them, we express our true and complete confidence in their ability to find their own solution. We don't abandon them. Instead, we say, "I trust you'll know what's right for you. I'm here to cheer you on and to help if you get really stuck."

The boundary is our limit of that support. There are all kinds of support options, along a wide spectrum: advice, connections, money—all the way to decision-making and taking over full control. The more we let whomever we love figure out their own stuff, the more heart voice power they'll generate for themselves. Loving with detachment is how we stay out of the Control Factory. If we trust that the people we love can sort out their own shit, they'll be far more inclined to do just that. When we treat them accordingly and expect them to be strong, healthy, and resilient, we give them the courage to rise to that challenge. And we give them the advantage of growing confident in their ability to succeed and navigate their own shitstorms.

> The more we let whomever we love figure out their
> own stuff, the more heart voice power
> they'll generate for themselves.

The Bottom Line About Boundaries

None of us are responsible for how people act. Or how they react. To anything. It's also not our duty to try to control their perspective. For sure, we'll make a bigger effort for the people we love to understand us. But, whenever we change, some people won't like it. They're used to us behaving in a predictable way, and they'll probably take steps to convince us to stay that way—especially if they're also listening to the town voices. It's human nature.

The good news is, we don't have to let them drag us back into Victimtown. The people who are tuned in to their own heart voice will support us and champion us on with the same loving detachment we offer to them. If you'd like to learn more about boundaries and loving detachment, Melody Beattie is my favorite expert on the topic. She's written many books about this, all of which I highly recommend, such as *Codependent No More* and *The Language of Letting Go.*

CHAPTER 24

Courage Is Learnable

The two hardest tests on the spiritual road are the patience to wait for the right moment and the courage not to be disappointed with what we encounter.

—*Paulo Coelho*, Veronika Decides to Die

Courage and fear are not mutually exclusive. Whenever we're being brave, we're also usually (at least a little bit) afraid. That's natural. It's also an opportune time for the town voices to pipe up. What if, instead, we embraced fear? What if we viewed our fears as an opportunity to learn and practice courage? It's our fears that provide the chance for growth and new insights. Which makes having fears and insecurities actually a good thing. Without the experience of overcoming our fears, our prospects of becoming a better human would be greatly diminished. There's a satisfaction in our growth and transformation and a pride in ourselves that isn't attainable any other way. There's also much joy available in the process. Each and every time we do a bit better and gain a little ground, we increase our heart voice power.

How each of us defines and integrates courage into our lives is fluid and extremely varied. Some people consider courage only to be acts of grand bravery, like fighting off a cougar to save your child, but I think it takes more courage to talk back to the town voices. The kind of courage that's required to leave Victimtown may feel every bit as extreme as a Herculean effort to fight a wild cougar. The way we each think about courage is a reflection of our unique experiences, which have shaped how we see the world. No two are the same. What's easy for some people takes tremendous courage for others. Please, let's remove judgment about this too. The one thing that everyone has in common when it comes to courage is that the foundation upon which our courage is built is supplied by our heart voice.

Intrinsic Courage

Here's what I believe is the ultimate definition of courage:

> **Intrinsic courage**
> **is our ability to view**
> **every past experience,**
> **every current situation, and**
> **every person involved**
> **with love and compassion.**

After coming up with this, I thought I was pretty smart. It sounded representative of all that I'd learned. Honorable, too. Then I put it to the test in my own life and, well, it wasn't as natural or easy as I hoped. Theoretically, I believe in it with my whole heart, yet there are times that I still have to remind myself of its merits. I'm committed to it, though. I practice as much as I can, because I know firsthand of its transformational power.

We were all born with an unlimited amount of love and compassion. We may be out of practice putting it to good use, but it's there inside all of us. That's why it's called intrinsic. Courage and our heart voice work together, hand in hand. They're faithful partners conceived to inspire, support, and enhance each other. Shit will happen, and we'll be challenged (sometimes immensely) to find a grain of love or compassion for the people involved or for the circumstances. When this occurs, our two greatest tools are curiosity and time.

Certain things are hard to let go of, especially fear. The Boss tells us that the situation will spin out of control and be a complete disaster if we don't manage every single thing and everyone involved. I was especially susceptible to those messages when it came to my kids. There were times I was so afraid of what might happen to them that I manipulated and enforced my will upon my kids. There were also things I was too afraid to do or say. Not understanding loving detachment resulted in a few situations around which I still hold deep regrets. I continue to practice intrinsic courage for myself. Because we can't change what happened, my heart voice confirms that I did the best I could, with the resources I had available at the time. I believe that's true for all of us, always.

What's hard to see in moments of fear is that spinning out of control can go in *any* direction. Spinning out of control can also produce a positive direction beyond our wildest dreams. Everyone and everything are entitled to spin their own way. We all deserve our own trajectory in life. When we let go of our need to control, it takes the pressure off. We can relax and enjoy the ride. This is happiness.

The best thing about intrinsic courage (this combo of heart voice power and courage) is that together, they make it possible for us to have *complete trust in all outcomes*. Together, they provide the support for us to let go of our fear. Together, they foster optimism. When our motivations and actions are based in love, it's possible to find everything we yearn for. Forgiveness can't help but flow naturally when we're able to embrace intrinsic courage. It's how we rewrite our stories, too.

Intrinsic courage makes it possible for us to
have *complete trust in all outcomes.*

We can embrace and practice intrinsic courage in the multiple small decisions and choices we make every day. We can reach for intrinsic courage in the pause when shit happens or any time afterward when we're facing difficulties.

The greatest thing about intrinsic courage is that, inevitably, it leads us to understand the role that every experience, situation, and person played to create an opportunity for us to learn, heal, and find joy. Our gratitude for these experiences allows us to conclude that forgiveness is actually unnecessary. I believe that our collective ability to embrace intrinsic courage when we're in pain has the power to change our world.

I'm daring to hope for a chance to forgive whomever is responsible for my Aunt Lynda's death. I might need some help with this. Having the courage to view them with love and compassion will be tough. But I'm gonna trust that I'll figure out how to get curious enough, with a strong heart voice, to do just that when the opportunity arrives.

Trust in All Outcomes

Letting go isn't always easy, but if we want out of Victimtown, it's something we've gotta do. You'll know in your heart whatever it is you need to let go of. It could be people, beliefs, environments, coping mechanisms, worry, or control, or something else. For me it was mostly about letting go of control. The only way I could do that was to grab onto something else. Because I worked at the Control Factory for so long, I needed something to be tethered to. To help myself let go, I grabbed onto complete trust in all outcomes—a faith that the universe has my back. This is what I count on to provide the outcomes for my highest and best good, even if that includes a shitty, hard life lesson or three.

Letting go of our old patterns and behaviors takes courage. We like what's comfortable and familiar, so it's normal to fear change. And the town voices will underscore our fears by telling us we're better off with a situation we know because worse possibilities await. The thing is, though, the universe can't figure things out for us, unless we trust it to do so. And if our situation is already pretty good, we won't enjoy even better circumstances until we trust enough to let go and embrace the unknown.

Worry is eradicated when we have complete trust in all outcomes. Ultimately, it no longer matters what the world throws at us because our heart voice will provide guidance and our courage will provide strength. We stop striving to control people and circumstances. We own our stories through love and compassion for ourselves. And we're able to process our own anger by viewing others with love and compassion. The Denial Trails no longer hold any perks, because our hearts are now strong enough to handle the most intolerable issues.

It no longer matters what the world throws at us
because our heart voice will provide guidance and
our courage will provide strength.

Maya Angelou famously said, "We delight in the beauty of the butterfly, but rarely admit the changes it has gone through to achieve that beauty." I love this quote because it invites compassion for ourselves as we also go through changes.

Impatience often leads us to abandon our trust in an outcome when things don't happen when we want them to or when we expect that they should. Let's not forget that timelines are issued by a town voice. An unwanted or surprising outcome can also derail our trust. Let's not forget that our trust must be placed in ALL outcomes, not just the specific ones we're focused on. Our hearts are a direct conduit to the universe. Trusting in all outcomes requires us to believe that we are always in the right place, doing the right thing at the right time.

I showed courage that day running home from school with a bursting bladder. My courage wasn't as much about my fear of leaving the group as it was about viewing myself with love and compassion when I got home and melted. Remember, intrinsic courage isn't just about others; it's for us first!

CHAPTER 25

Victimtown vs. Freedomville

The difference between school and life?
In school, you're taught a lesson and
then given a test. In life, you're given a
test that teaches you a lesson.
—*Tom Bodett*

About a year after I left The Place, someone I loved dearly was struggling. Like, a lot. They were in a really bad place. The town voices showed up and started to get LOUD. I was so afraid for them that I began to imagine disastrous outcomes. And I started to plot what I needed to do to fix it. Panic was right around the corner.

Too bad you don't have a bottle of wine. Now would be the perfect time. Remember how good it felt? Just a glass, at least take the edge off . . .

No, I don't want wine. I haven't had a drink in close to a year.

Wine would make it all go away. It's only fifteen minutes to town.

Wait. There's some old weed cookies in the freezer.

I open the freezer to look at them. Three medium-sized cookies in a Ziploc that my friend Gary made last year. I take one out and feel it. It's hard as a rock.

A ten-second zap will cure that.

I just need a short reprieve. Just one evening to not worry about anything. To stop this voice from yattering in my head. I zap the cookie and have a taste.

That was a pretty small bite. Probably won't do much.

I think back to the conversation we had when he gave me the cookies as I take another little bite. He said that he wasn't sure how strong they were, but he'd eaten half of one, and he'd let me know. Squinting my eyes, I look up at the ceiling for answers. . . . Did I ever hear back from him? What did he say? Concluding that I was not gonna remember, I wonder if I should give him a call.

Oh, come on! Finish the cookie and chill out.

So I do.

It'll be fine.

It was a Wednesday. Euchre night. My dad and I were going next door for our usual evening of four fun-filled card games and witty banter with our neighbors Wendy and Steve. My dad had a late lunch and wasn't interested in dinner. All I'd eaten since noon was the cookie, so I grab a bag of tortilla chips and some salsa, and I drive us over because, even with a flashlight, the forest trail between our houses is treacherous in the pitch black of night.

I'm starting to feel the effects when we arrive—a calm and welcome relaxation of my body and mind. We take our seats at the kitchen table where the nearby woodstove has made it cozy and warm.

Yep. This is what I'm talkin' about. . . .

I get euchred once and lose the first game. Then the fire gets stoked, and we switch partners. By the middle of game two, I'm having trouble remembering what's trump. And not just with each hand. I'm having trouble remembering what's trump with every card led!

Concentrate, Liz! You can't keep asking what's trump. They're gonna wonder what's going on with you. Boy, it's getting really warm in here. . . .

I play terribly, but I muddle through. I lose again. Per standard procedure, we take a break after the second game so my dad and Wendy can go outside to smoke. Cigarettes. Steve puts another log in the woodstove and says, "Are you okay? You look really tired."

Oh my God! My eyelids weigh, like, a thousand pounds!

"I'm good. I've just been dealing with some stuff lately," I said.

You need to explain your eyes, stupid.

"And I am kinda tired," I add.

The door opens and the smokers return. Game three requires new partners again. New partners require a seat change. But I've got a problem. My body has become one with the chair, and I seriously doubt my ability to perform this basic task. In fact, I'm terrified to even try, so I don't. My friends organize the seating themselves and unknowingly solve my dilemma.

Phew. That was close.

Then I get the first jack. It's my deal. The dexterity required for me to gather the cards into a pile takes a hellacious effort. I watch my hands like they belong to someone else as I attempt to shuffle and deal the cards. I stop twice in the middle of dealing to count how many cards I've passed out. And I giggle to myself. Out loud.

I think they're staring at you. Don't make eye contact.

Barely able to maintain the motor skills necessary to hold the fan of cards, I grapple to pick out a single card and lay it on the table. I renege multiple times. Obviously, I lose game three too. I am beyond wasted.

And then I start to feel nauseous.

It must be 130 degrees in here. I need to splash some water on my face. Preferably ice-cold. You'll have to stand up and walk to do that. Shit.

The nausea gets worse.

You have to get up. Now. One, two, three, go!

A little wobbly, but with determination, I stand and gather my wits.

With immense concentration, I place one foot in front of the other and make it to the washroom. Just in time. It feels like hours before I'm able to find some Listerine and rinse my mouth. I slink back to the kitchen.

You're a stupid asshole, Liz. You're embarrassing yourself.

"Steve," I said. "I think I need you to drive me home." I turn my head.

"Wendy," I said. "I think I need you to help me put my coat and boots on." And then.

"Hey, Dad," I said. "I think I need to go to bed."

The next day, the voices in my head confirmed my return to Victimtown. Well aware that I listened to a Dirtbag and spent my evening on the Denial Trails, the balance of the following day was wasted lying on the couch, half stoned, regretting how I misjudged and mishandled the pause. It was all I could do to keep the Maître D's yacking to a minimum.

Everyone maintains the right to visit Victimtown. We might go there for ourselves or for someone else. We can go deliberately or by accident. At least now, we'll have an awareness of where we are, how we got there, and what we need to do to get out.

A circumstance might arise where the Boss attempts to recruit you for a special assignment. She'll offer promises of a big paycheck, a great benefit plan, or a lifelong salary. Enticements like that—especially when the special assignment involves someone we love—can lure us into taking the job of rescuing them. The mission, however, will require a trip to Victimtown. It won't be an easy decision, and all I can say about it is this: Listen carefully to distinguish the voices in your head and pay attention to all the intel delivered by your feelings. Taking the time to uncover and explore your true motivations will help to discern whether the recommended action is coming from your heart or the Boss.

If it's your heart voice advising you to visit someone, you'll have a different agenda in Victimtown than if you're acting under the Boss's direction. Someone might genuinely need your support. If people in Victimtown want what we're offering, we can help. We can guide them, but we can't pull anyone out of Victimtown. No one leaves unless and until they're ready. If we take them by force, odds are they'll go right back the first chance they get.

Extended Visits

Even with awareness, visits to Victimtown for someone other than ourselves have risks. We arrive with no time to waste, and we usually know where to find whomever we're looking for. People in Victimtown tend to have a favorite spot. Maybe they're at the Guilt & Shame Café. Our good intentions to have a short visit can quickly go awry. They usually won't be ready to leave. They're hungry. They wanna talk. We think to ourselves, "Okay, I'll just stay for a quick bite, and then we can leave together," but they've got a different agenda. They want to relax with a few drinks first. Then appetizers, a main course, dessert, and then, yup, more drinks.

It takes a lot of courage to get up and leave Victimtown. But if we don't, we'll find ourselves sitting in a dark corner talking about how awful life is. Before long, we too are feeling super shitty about ourselves and our brutal and pointless lives, and then in our misery, we forget about trying to help them. The Maître D' stops by to chat and commiserate, and we drink some more. . . .

At some point, hopefully, we think, "Man, I gotta stop doing this." I'm not saying that abandoning your friends is the answer. We can pull up a chair outside the café and let them know they're not alone. We can listen with empathy and tell them they're loved. We can wait for them and be there to help them leave, but they have to make the decision to leave themselves.

Nobody likes to see anyone stuck in the Sorrow Swampland, and we're only human to want to help them. It's a good intention, but most of us aren't qualified to pull them out, no matter how strong we are, no matter how much we want to. The Monster has a hold on people. If they're stuck, they are stuck. The muck will not thin out until their own heart voice leads the way. What we can do is sit on the bench nearby. They'll know we're close. My good friend Edy Nathan is a psychotherapist and grief doula. Her book *It's Grief: The Dance of Self-Discovery through Trauma and Loss* is an excellent resource. We can offer to bring help to friends ensnared by the Monster. But until the people we love are ready to leave, that's all we can do.

For their own reasons, at whatever place suits them, lots of people don't want to be alone in Victimtown. Misery loves company. If we know anyone like that, we're at risk of getting dragged into an extended stay. I'm not talking about the people who want hand-holding support; the folks we need to be wary of are the ones who want us to be Thelma to their Louise. In our hearts, we know better. It takes boundaries and practice to stand up to these peeps because the more desperate they are, the more convincing they can be.

The Gifts in Victimtown

Visiting Victimtown is unavoidable. If we didn't return to these places, it would mean our souls have finished evolving and we've learned all the life lessons that exist on earth. Nobody's learned *all* the lessons, at least nobody I know! Our new level of awareness and understanding enables us to notice when we've returned to a behavior that we're trying to change or avoid because now we recognize that we're in Victimtown.

Sometimes it's a test to see if we've fully integrated the lesson that brought us here the last time. It's a huge confidence boost to come back into town and know what to do. I called my best friend, Deb, the day after euchre night and recounted the events. After several minutes of deep belly laughing, she said, "Yeah, you spent the evening on the trail—and then breakfast at the Guilt & Shame Café. Sounds like you had lunch there too. Is that really where you want to eat dinner?" BAM. She called me out in a way that made me realize what I was doing but didn't make me feel embarrassed or bad about it. I laughed back and planned some radical self-care for the rest of the day. Deb's one of the smartest people I know.

We can play the same awareness game with others. Victimtown—and all the places there—gives us a new language to use when we're talking about hard and vulnerable mental health issues. It may require mutual agreement ahead of time, depending on your relationship, but using the names of the places eliminates the stigma associated with being there. If we happen to visit Victimtown, the sooner we know where we are, the sooner we can leave. We can also have more empowering and supportive conversations with our friends:

> "Hey, I didn't know you took a job at the Control Factory! What's really going on?"

> "Why are you at the Guilt & Shame Café? I thought you were avoiding that place. How can I help?"

> "Come on, let's get out of the Ego Arena."

> "I know it's hard, but the Dirtbags are just gonna hand that issue right back to you when you leave the Denial Trails. What support do you need to face it?"

> "Sorry I didn't call you back. I fueled up at the Anger Gas Station and ended up in the Sorrow Swampland. It's been a tough weekend."

> "How am I? Well, I'll tell ya. I've been parked in the Resentment Parking Lot all weekend, and my voice is hoarse from all my grudge-telling."

> "The Dirtbags keep giving me bad directions, and I'm trying to find my way off this shitty Denial Trails system. Can you help me?"

There's no need to squirm when we find ourselves in Victimtown. Admitting and talking about it is healthy for us. It's a lighter and less vulnerable way to let the people we love into our world. It's an easier way to express what's going on with us. It gives people the information they need to support us, and it's a casual way to ask for help. It also provides the insights we need to support the people we care about.

Victimtown is also where we go until we're able to process our pain. We spend time at one place or another until we're ready to heal. Very often, the realization of where we are is enough to shift our perspective so we can begin to take steps toward Freedomville.

Even after we've healed our past traumas and hurts, there are always more lessons. Always. Some new lessons won't require a visit to Victimtown because now we know how it all works, but many will. It's fair to expect that the hardest lessons might land us in at least one of the places, for a little while anyway. That's okay. Our lessons last a lifetime. That's why we're here. That's why Victimtown exists: to offer us gifts.

Freedomville Awaits

Instinctively, you've always known what it takes to live in Freedomville: heart voice power and intrinsic courage. You were born with both. Neither is effortless or always straightforward, but they're a sure-fire way to find the peace, love, freedom, and joy that we all yearn for. Practicing radical self-care, forgiveness, and boundaries provide us with the strength to maintain our heart voice power and to act with intrinsic courage when shit gets real. Your complete trust in all outcomes provides solace through the worst hardships. This is how to navigate shitstorms.

It takes heart voice power and intrinsic courage to
live in Freedomville. You were born with both.

Freedomville is available for everyone. There's an easy flow to life here. We feel fulfilled and happy. The chaos in our heads is gone. Love is in the air.

While I can't speak for my family, I've only recently processed my feelings about my childhood, and I've (mostly) ditched the three shitty beliefs. My heart voice rules the roost more days than not, but I still have my moments as I continue to work on the practical stuff. I'm a total newbie in the boundary department, and it's hard for me.

Intrinsic courage is my biggest source of inspiration, and it's what I come back to when I don't know what to do or which way to go. I know that love and compassion will keep me from getting lost again, but applying it to some of the shit that happens sure isn't a walk in the park.

Lynda was in my life for a reason. I need and want to honor her. Lynda's life journey provided the circumstances necessary to give me the opportunity to embark on the long expedition required to reclaim my heart voice and, ultimately, to teach intrinsic courage. And maybe, just maybe, if I'm able to succeed at that, answers will arrive, and we'll finally know what happened to her. When I meet the person responsible for her death, it will be the ultimate test of my intrinsic courage. And I'll need your help.

Let's start a movement! I invite you to put the companion guidebook to good use, to cultivate your own heart voice, to love yourself without limits or conditions and to practice intrinsic courage. As you trust in all outcomes, whatever you yearn for will eventually arrive. In the meantime, I hope you'll find it easier to navigate any shitstorms that come your way.

From the bottom of my heart, thank you for your time to read this book. For inspiration, new offerings, or to shoot me a message about how you're doing, you'll find me at www.lizlongwrites.com.

My Heart Voice Plea

As of this writing, at least one person has been living with the weight of Lynda's death on their conscience for over fifty-four years. That's about 20,000 mornings (and counting) that they have woken up and remembered what happened.

I imagine they are exhausted and yearning for peace.

My personal message to them is this:

> *I think about you every day. I now see your participation in the gift of my awakening. I know you are suffering. That traumatic, and perhaps accidental, night in 1968 sent many people to Victimtown, including you and me. I lived there for a long time, but I'm grateful to have finally left having reclaimed my heart voice power. With love and compassion, I would like to offer you a road out. Please . . . listen to your heart, come forward, and take my hand.*

And to anyone, anywhere, who may know something about what happened to Lynda:

No information is insignificant. Don't be afraid to speak up.
It's not too late to do the right thing. You can do it anonymously.
Please come forward and release the pain of your secret.

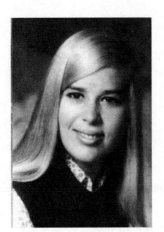

LYNDA MARY LOUISE WHITE

Born: March 25, 1949
Last seen: November 13, 1968
(age 19)
Body discovered: May 9, 1973
Case #: 955-10-101-1996

To report information:
Call CRIMESTOPPERS 1-800-222-8477.
Or visit: https://www.canadiancrimestoppers.org.

Acknowledgments

I am so very fortunate to have people who accept me and love me and who are always there to support me on this wild journey called life. I'm at a loss of words to describe my gratitude and love for Deb Bakti, who steadfastly stood by me at my lowest and who dropped everything to drive hundreds of miles and put me on a plane to The Place. Honestly, this "Acknowledgments" section is the hardest part of the whole book. Damn. I'm gonna cry again (tears of joy though). I'll tell y'all more in person. If I've overlooked anyone, please accept my heartfelt apology. My memory truly is still very shitty, but I'm working on it. It's my great privilege to both navigate shitstorms and revel in the calm and joy of Freedomville with Kyle Wilson, Katherine Rammo, Adam Wilson, River, Andy Long, Greg Long, Karen Lloyd, Lynda White, Joan White, Heather White, Nana, Bampa and the entire White Family, Edy Nathan, Debbie DiMascio, Simona Dutka, Deanna Louise, Tara Stamp, the Tulips, Jace, Jenny, Lex, Ed, Yon, Sunil, Lisa, Sam, and all the staff at The Place.

Producing this book was so much more *everything* than I imagined. I could never have done it alone! My heartfelt thanks for the encouragement and expertise of Deborah Bakti, AJ Harper, Jennifer MacMillan, Karen Graham, Charlene Lite, along with all of my advance readers and everyone at Greenleaf Book Group.

Lastly, I'd like to acknowledge all the people who I thought did me wrong, treated me like shit, or hurt me in some way. My responses landed me in one (or many) of the places in Victimtown. In your own way, each of you gave me a profound gift—a chance to redeem my heart voice and practice intrinsic courage. Most of you paid a personal price for that, and I hope you'll accept my gratitude. I honor your role in shaping my life. Without you, I wouldn't be where, or who, I am today.

Liz is grateful to live, work, and play on the unceded lands of the shíshálh (Sechelt) Nation and the nearby Sḵwx̱wú7mesh Úxwumixw (Squamish Nation) with her heartfelt acknowledgment of the deep injustices Native people have endured over the centuries.

Notes

Introduction

1. "Why Words Die: How to Keep Lexical Treasures from Keeling Over," *The Economist*, March 4, 2017, https://www.economist.com/books-and -arts/2017/03/04/why-words-die.

Chapter 2

1. "Fast Facts: Preventing Adverse Childhood Experiences," Centers for Disease Control and Prevention, last modified April 6, 2022, https://www.cdc.gov/ violenceprevention/aces/fastfact.html.

2. Bruce D. Perry and Oprah Winfrey, *What Happened to You?: Conversations on Trauma, Resilience, and Healing* (New York: Flatiron Books, 2021).

Chapter 4

1. Perry and Winfrey, *What Happened to You?*

Chapter 6

1. "EMDR: Eye Movement Desensitization and Reprocessing," WebMD, last modified November 6, 2021, https://www.webmd.com/mental-health/emdr -what-is-it#:~:text=Eye%20movement%20desensitization%20and%20 reprocessing%20(EMDR)%20is%20a%20fairly%20new,traumatic%20 stress%20disorder%20(PTSD).

Chapter 8

1. Jane Sims, "Box of Clues Found in Late Cop's Home May Help Solve Cold Cases," *Toronto Sun*, March 22, 2014, https://torontosun.com/2014/03/22/box-of-clues-found-in-late-cops-home-may-help-solve-cold-cases.

Chapter 14

1. Jonathan Frostick, "So I Had a Heart Attack . . .," LinkedIn, April, 2021, https://www.linkedin.com/feed/update/urn:li:activity:6787207960864014336/.

Chapter 15

1. Emily Maroutian, *The Book of Relief: Passages and Exercises to Relieve Negative Emotion and Create More Ease in the Body* (Independently published, 2021).

Chapter 17

1. Brené Brown, *Daring Greatly: How the Courage to Be Vulnerable Transforms the Way We Live, Love, Parent, and Lead* (New York: Avery, 2015).

Chapter 19

1. "IASP Announces Revised Definition of Pain," IASP, July 16, 2020, https://www.iasp-pain.org/publications/iasp-news/iasp-announces-revised-definition-of-pain/.

2. Dr. Bradley Nelson, *The Emotion Code: How to Release Your Trapped Emotions for Abundant Health, Love, and Happiness* (New York: St. Martin's Essentials, 2019).

3. "Deaths from Excessive Alcohol Use in the United States," Centers for Disease Control and Prevention, last modified July 6, 2022, https://www.cdc.gov/alcohol/features/excessive-alcohol-deaths.html#:~:text=More%20than%20140%2C000%20people%20die,how%20you%20can%20take%20action.

4. Annie Grace, *This Naked Mind: Alcohol Control: Find Freedom, Discover Happiness & Change Your Life* (New York: Avery, 2015).

5. Jeff Weiner, "The Importance of Scheduling Nothing," LinkedIn, April 3, 2013, https://www.linkedin.com/pulse/20130403215758-22330283-the-importance-of-scheduling-nothing/.

6. Britta K. Hölzel et al., "Mindfulness Practice Leads to Increases in Regional Brain Gray Matter Density," *Psychiatry Research: Neuroimaging* 191, no. 1 (January 2011): 36–43, https://doi.org/10.1016/j.pscychresns.2010.08.006.

7. Emily Fletcher, "The M Word: Meditation to Uplevel Your Life," Mindvalley, October 9, 2019, https://www.mindvalley.com/mword/.

Chapter 21

1. Eva Selhub, "Nutritional Psychiatry: Your brain on Food," Harvard Health Blog, *Harvard Health Publishing*, September 18, 2022, https://www.health.harvard.edu/blog/nutritional-psychiatry-your-brain-on-food-201511168626.

2. Angela Jacques et al., "The Impact of Sugar Consumption on Stress Driven, Emotional and Addictive Behaviors," *Neuroscience & Biobehavioral Reviews* 103 (August 2019): 178–199, https://doi.org/10.1016/j.neubiorev.2019.05.021.

3. Julia Rodriguez, "CDC Declares Sleep Disorders a Public Health Epidemic," The Sleep Blog, Advance Sleep Medicine Services, Inc., accessed November 9, 2022, https://www.sleepdr.com/the-sleep-blog/cdc-declares-sleep-disorders-a-public-health-epidemic/.

4. Earl S. Ford, Timothy J. Cunningham, and Janet B. Croft, "Trends in Self-Reported Sleep Duration among US Adults from 1985 to 2012," *SLEEP* 38, no. 5 (May 2015): 829–832, doi: 10.5665/sleep.4684.

5. Ying He et al., "The Transcriptional Repressor DEC2 Regulates Sleep Length in Mammals," *Science* 325, no. 5942 (August 2009): 866–870, doi: 10.1126/science.1174443.

6. Roger S. Ulrich, "View Through a Window May Influence Recovery from Surgery," *Science* 224, no. 4647 (April 1984): 420–421, doi: 10.1126/science.6143402.

Chapter 22

1. "Forgiveness," Wikimedia Foundation, last modified September 18, 2022, 10:59, https://en.wikipedia.org/wiki/Forgiveness.

About the Author

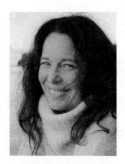 **Liz Long** is one of 8 billion human beings on Earth. No better or worse than any other, she's finding her way in her own time, as we all do. She continues to make mistakes, to learn and heal, and find more joy.

Liz is a thinker, feeler, and communicator with a mission to guide and encourage people to live with intrinsic courage. Her **Heart Voice Power Plan©** helps people learn to love themselves without limits or conditions, which makes intrinsic courage not only possible but attainable.

Liz has two adult sons, a cat, and a granddog. She lives in Sechelt, British Columbia, with her dad. You can connect with her at www. lizlongwrites.com.